INSTINCTIVE
NUTRITION

INSTINCTIVE NUTRITION

Severen L. Schaeffer

CELESTIALARTS
Berkeley, California

CELESTIAL ARTS
P.O. Box 7327
Berkeley, California 94707

Cover photo by Ben Aisles
Cover design by Ken Scott
Text design by Paul Reed
Typography by HMS Typography, Inc.

Library of Congress Cataloging-in-Publication Data

Schaeffer, Severen L.
    Instinctive nutrition.

    Includes Index.
    1. Diet therapy.   I. Title.   [DNLM: 1. Food Habits—
popular works.   2. Health.   3. Instinct—popular works.
4. Nutrition—popular works.   QU 145 S294i]
RM216.S356 1988   615.8'54   87-18248
ISBN 0-89087-502-2

Manufactured in the United States of America

First Printing, 1987

1 2 3 4 5 – 91 90 89 88 87

Reader
Please Note

The recommendations in this book are not intended as medical advice. Before undertaking instinctive nutrition, particularly if you are under medical supervision or are taking medication for a specific physical problem, you are advised to consult with your physician.

If you decide to take up eating by instinct and find it isn't working for you, then stop. The intent of this book is to point out things you may do, not things you *must* do. The book explains that food can constitute a potent therapeutic tool in many cases, but this should not be construed as an incitement to abandon medical treatment. Particularly with respect to medical drugs, before making any changes, consult with the physician who prescribed them.

It must be understood that a book cannot substitute for the personal guidance and supervision that are often necessary to help a beginner recognize toxin-laden food and properly select food for maximum effectiveness. For this reason, although the author has made every effort to provide clear practical guidelines, he cannot assume responsibility for any interpretation and use the reader may make of them. If you use the methods explained here, you should clearly understand that you are doing so at your own risk.

— Severen L. Schaeffer

Contents

PART II: FOOD, HEALTH, AND ILLNESS

PART III: DOING IT YOURSELF

Foreword

by Norman Shealy, M.D., Ph.D.

In no aspect of human behavior is there greater variety, controversy, and dogma than there is in the field of nutrition. For many years, John Tobby pushed the idea of a totally raw or uncooked diet, and yet, he died in his 70's of cancer of the prostate. Anne Wigmore has also pushed a diet that is largely raw. Nutrition varies from the average American diet, which most intelligent people would admit is terrible, to the Macrobiotic diet, the Pritikin diet, the Haas Eat To Win diet, and the McDougal Plan. These latter four all have a great deal of cooked food but are primarily five to ten percent fat and mostly complex carbohydrate-containing diets. Proponents all make a number of claims for their respective diets.

When I first heard from Severen Schaeffer about *Anopson* nutrition and the statements that he was making about its efficiency, I found it intriguing and somewhat hard to believe. Fortunately, I had an opportunity to sponsor a workshop on Anopson, or instinctive nutrition, therapy. My own reactions to this way of eating were fascinating, as were those of other attendees at this small workshop. I consumed huge quantities of plums and honey among other delicacies with a variety of reactions to tell me when I was satiated. I tried to continue eating this way and found it difficult, primarily because I could not find raw fish or beef that I was willing to eat. I think it would be difficult to practice the method correctly without these two foods.

Several other attendees at that workshop, however, have stayed on it to a greater or lesser extent with remarkably encouraging results. One dentist who had had severe psoriasis and micronychia has reported marked improvement within a few months. He had tried many other treatments without success previously. Increased energy and sense of well-being have been reported uniformly by those attempting the diet, most with mild modifications.

The video tapes of individuals in France who have had the optimal Anopson diet are as impressive as anything I have ever seen in clinical medicine. I have certainly seen enough in those video tapes and in the response of those individuals attending the Anopson workshop to convince me that Instinctive Nutrition deserves extensive, careful, scientific study. For those individuals who have significant illnesses, I cannot think of a better and safer approach than Anopsotherapy or Instinctive Nutrition.

— Norman Shealy, M.D., Ph.D.
Director, Shealy Pain & Health Rehabilitation Institute
Founding President, American Holistic Medical Association

Preface

Mankind's long road from darkness to light has been a pave-as-you-go affair, subject to washouts. It is not clear which end we stand nearer to. Periodically, bandits post signs saying "Nothing Exists Beyond This Point" — and proceed to rob travellers who are foolish enough to stop. But the builders are many, so the road has many branches. Some of them wind toward nowhere, but are so wide and well built that they appear to be direct routes. Others do go forward, but on paths so faint and narrow they can hardly.be seen, so that no normal person with common sense will use them. Only abnormal people with *un*common sense venture forth upon these ways.

Late in the 15th century, a Genoese navigator and opportunist named Christopher Columbus advanced the *absurd* proposition that one might reach the east by sailing west. It took him nearly a decade to find a sponsor for such a voyage, for it was *common knowledge* at the time that the world was flat, and that vessels sailing too far from shore would fall off the edge. Although more by chance than by intent, this outrageous idea led to the discovery of the New World.

Some 150 years later, an Italian mathematician, Galileo Galilei, advanced another absurd proposition. The earth, said he, revolves around the sun. It was absurd because *everyone knew* that the earth was the center of the universe. But it was dangerous as well, because if it was true, it was a threat to the power of the church and other vested interests of the day. The Inquisition tried Galileo and shut him away, but failed to repress a discovery whose time had come.

Human beings are by nature *believers*. We conduct our affairs according to whatever representations of "reality" we take to be "facts." We value what we "know" to be "true," and may argue or even fight to keep our convictions intact. We are human, and paradoxically, intelligent but not "dumb" enough to be *wise*. Like monkeys, we are capable of fighting over bananas . . . unlike monkeys who will only do so when there *are* some.

The story that follows leads far from the mainstream of current belief, but must ultimately change its course. You may be tempted to dismiss it as "merely an interesting notion," and by expressing your certainty that we cannot be sure of *anything* (except, of course, your certainty), you can accomplish that. Then again, you may want to take it seriously. But how to do so? If multi-million-dollar research projects, employing thousands of biologists, chemists, etc., in laboratories so sophisticated that a degree is required even to understand their purpose — if these men and women have thus far failed to find a cure for arthritis, cancer, schizophrenia or the common cold . . . is it possible to take seriously the suggestion that the answers are not to be found in science at all, but rather in human "instinct"?

Hardly.

Because as usual, we are not really prepared to accept ideas that are alien to our beliefs. If they are only slightly unorthodox and we have kept an open mind, we may grant them some space within our system of understanding. But suppose they are genuine heresy?

The theses set forth here are basic to human well-being. Like Columbus's, they will elicit objections and warnings — and lead to the discovery of new landscapes. Like Galileo's, they will endanger the Established Order. They will be obvious to children, perplexing to adults, anathema to cooks . . . and for many, nothing less than a godsend.

PART I
THE HUMAN INSTINCT FOR FOOD

Introduction

In the early fall of 1983, an erudite and somewhat defensive gentleman by the name of Guy-Claude Burger came to give a talk at the School of Medicine of the University of Paris, where I teach. He had reputedly cured himself with food of a cancer, and was going to tell us how he had done it.

I found his exposé fascinating. Informed by his physicians that medicine held no hope for his cancer (a lymphoblastic sarcoma of the larynx), he had, at age 26, isolated himself on a farm in his native Switzerland and set forth to heal himself. Convinced that the artifacts of civilization were responsible for his "disease of civilization," he decided to "get back to nature" as closely as possible and took to living without electricity, phones, heating – or commercial foodstuffs. Over a period of several months his cancer receded and eventually disappeared.

Burger was a physicist, but an accomplished cellist as well, a member of a Swiss chamber orchestra. In order to avoid restaurants while on tour, he carried fresh fruit and vegetables in his suitcase. This meant he was frequently eating the same items, and his curiosity was aroused by a strange phenomenon: at one meal, cabbage would taste good, while at another, it would bite his tongue. And subsequently it would taste good once again.

Experimenting further, Burger discovered that with foods in their native, original state — but not with cooked foods — the taste as well as the smell would go bad at some point. He concluded that human beings possessed a built-in instinctive mechanism that was telling them when they had fulfilled their need for a particular food. Putting this into practice, he discovered that sick people could often recover rapidly, even from severe illnesses, once they began trusting their senses, eating a variety of raw, original foods.

It was apparent that Burger had touched upon something fundamental. He had conducted numerous experiments, over nearly 20 years, but had failed to document them fully. His theoretical explanations sometimes raised eyebrows, and some of his claims seemed extravagant. But his innovative thesis that men were genetically adapted only to foods in their original native state seemed sound, and a number of us became interested in knowing more. We suggested the system be called "Anopsology" to replace the "Instinctotherapy" label it had been going by.

When an Instinctive Nutrition center was finally opened in the fall of 1984, in an old chateau south of Paris, a few of us went there as observers. What we saw in some cases was truly astounding: people who had been ill or in pain for years, some of them medically "incurable," regaining their health with food. I have included some of their testimonials and case histories in this book.

Anopsotherapy obviously works — but *why*? The following pages attempt to answer that question. I have tried to formulate the answers in ways consistent with current knowledge in medicine, genetics, biochemistry, nutrition, etc. But I trust the reader will appreciate the fact that much of our understanding in these areas comes from the study of *abnormally* nourished people or from laboratory studies *in Vitro*. Anopsology will, I believe, cause us to question many assumptions in medicine and nutrition that we generally take for granted.

I would like to express my appreciation to Guy-Claude Burger for enabling me to live and work at the French National Anopsological Center for extended periods between 1984 and 1986, and for his patience and open-mindedness in replying to the endless questions, objections and observations I put to him. Thanks too, to Dr. Jean de Bonnefon, former clinic chief at Salpetrière hospital in Paris, who helped in obtaining and analyzing the case histories of former Anopsotherapy patients, and to Dr. Catherine Aimelet, consulting physician at the Center. Their comments are included along with commentaries from other physicians and from patients themselves. This material shows, I believe, that Anopsotherapy constitutes a major therapeutic technique, even though statistical data is as yet unavailable because the history of the discipline is so short.

I began personally to live Anopsologically near the end of 1983. Doing so cured me of smoking, tightened my gums so that my teeth no longer moved, ended a life-long history of colitis and ileitis, improved my vision, cured my allergy to cats, removed my cellulite, and left me in a better state of health than I had ever known, with an apparent general immunity to physical pain or infection. A growing number of people share my convictions as to its importance. Not a few among them, skeptical as I myself was at the outset, also became convinced of its fundamental validity from experiencing it for themselves.

This book is the first presentation of Anopsotherapy in the English language', and a first step to making it known and accessible in America. It is by no means "complete" and will require much amplification and amending as time goes on. It has several aims. If you are ill and suffering, it will show you a natural way to regain your health and alleviate your pain, if you will take the trouble to understand the principles involved and actually apply them. If you are among those responsible for raising, processing and serving food, it will, I hope, incite you to avoid methods that may harm those who eat that food. If you are a physician or other health professional, I hope it will inspire you to explore human dimensions that were never a part of your academic curriculum, so that you may truly help patients whom medicine would otherwise fail.

Severen L. Schaeffer
Paris, France

' Please see the bibliography at the end of this volume.

Chapter 1

Instinctive Nutrition: An Overview

Most people today are aware that nutrition plays a vital role in their health. You are probably concerned with eating a "balanced" diet containing sufficient minerals, vitamins, fibers, etc., to fill your needs. You are also probably a bit confused as to just exactly what "sufficient" might mean. At various times you may have tried one diet or another, one type of food supplement or another, one or another nutritional philosophy. The chances are that for a time, or to a degree, whatever you were doing made you feel more vital, or lose weight . . . and then, for some obscure reason, it didn't work so well any longer, or it became difficult or unsatisfying to keep up. Then you just forgot about dieting or supplements for awhile, until a new diet or formula caught your attention. Until this one did — except that it is neither a diet nor a formula.

Alternatively, you may at some point have adopted a system such as vegetarianism or macrobiotics, and decided that this was The Way, once and for all. If you are this sort of nutritional "true believer," be forewarned: Instinctive Nutrition will require you to forget your *beliefs* and attend to your *senses*, and if you are unwilling to attempt this, it will not work for you.

We are very literally what we eat. Food can make us healthy, but it can also make us sick, and it can kill us. Much of what we generally consume in quest of the former is doing the latter. It does so slowly, however, so we fail to recognize it. Once you have learned to eat by instinct, you will be able automatically to distinguish between foods that produce health and those that destroy it. Paradoxically, they are often one and the same, for "one man's meat is another man's poison" is more than an allegory. In a moment we will see how this is so.

Food can both produce disease and cure it, and we are going to discuss this at some length in order to give you a feeling for the processes involved. We will show you a method for preventing disease and healing it with foods selected by instinct. Its technical name is *Anopsotherapy*, also called "Instinctotherapy." It has been shown to be effective in curing even some conditions that are normally considered "incurable." It is based on the discovery that man is as fully endowed as any animal with a genetically determined alimentary instinct, and that his built-in programming can guide him to the food that will cure him and keep him well. It teaches us to use our senses to choose the nutrients our bodies truly need, free from restrictive precepts or recipes. It is emphatically *not* a diet.

The Greek word "Opson" means "prepared food." The "AN" prefix means "without" so that ANopson means "unprepared food." Here, however, "unprepared" should be understood as synonymous with "original," i.e., food *in the state in which it is found in nature.* A food that has been ground, frozen, cooked, mixed or otherwise denatured in any way does not fit this definition of *Anopson.* Fruits or vegetables bred by artificial selection and/or grown on chemical fertilizers, or animals fed hormones, mixed grains, etc., are not strictly *Anopson* by this definition (but are all too often the only kinds available.) Anopsology, or the "logic of Anopson," is the study of what happens when men and animals consume foods in their original, unmodified state, selecting them by instinctive sense-cues alone.

Anopsological (or Instinctive) Nutrition differs substantially from the nutritional philosophy of "Crudivorism," that already existed at the time of Socrates, and has become increasingly popular today. The idea that "raw food is good for us" is correct as far as it goes, but is inadequate and misses the point.

The human brain has been shown to be organized essentially on three levels. Its lowermost structures are known as the "reptilian brain," because they comprise our phylogenetic heritage from distant reptilian ancestors. These structures are common to all vertebrates, and organize basic survival behaviors: feeding, reproduction, fight/flight reactions, etc. These functions are automatic, built-in, and operate independently of learning from experience. They are what we commonly call *instincts*.

"Instincts" have been around a long time. The fossil record indicates that the simplest life forms appeared on earth roughly 2.5 billion years ago, and their evolution into cellular and multicellular organisms was very slow. Here and there mutations occured, which started new lineages leading to fish, lizards, birds, insects, etc. Fossil remains show that small mammals first appeared approximately 100 million years ago.

As they evolved along divergent developmental lines they gave rise to monkeys, apes, etc. (50 million years ago) and finally to *homo erectus*, who appeared about 5 million years into the past. Man's earliest use of fire for cooking dates back roughly 400,000 years. Agriculture and cattle-raising began only around 8,000 B.C.

If we were to imagine the course of evolution as a road 25 miles long, men would be coming into existence only 70 yards from the end, the discovery of cooking 25 feet from the end, and the development of agriculture about five inches before our time. Coca-Cola would appear roughly 1/200th of an inch into the past.

For nearly the whole length of this road, our predecessors ate only whatever they could find or catch, and ate it the way they found it. They necessarily chose their food the way any animal except man still does today: by smell and taste. If its smell and taste were attractive, they moved toward it; and if they were unattractive, they moved away. Human babies respond this way, and so do chimpanzees, our nearest genetic cousins. Neither possesses nutritional theories or taboos, or modifies his food before it goes in his mouth. Their responses are instinctive.

These instinctive responses are the fruit of evolution. Over millions of years, the process of natural selection ensured survival only for those species that were adapted to their environments. In biochemical terms, the survivors were those whose genetic codes (their DNA) had programmed them organismically to detect, select, ingest, digest and metabolize the kinds of available foods they needed to survive (as well as eliminate unuseable or toxic material that was inadvertently or unavoidably consumed at the same time). The survivors were also the ones who were programmed to avoid natural poisons.

It is thanks to their built-in, DNA-programmed sensory systems that bees are attracted to flowers, cows to grass, squirrels to nuts. The scheme of the universe, whatever it may be, was in play long before the emergence of the human neo-cortical capacity to analyze it . . . or tamper with it.

Is mankind genetically adapted to Coke? This question should not be taken lightly. The time-spans involved in evolutionary processes are enormous. Since the advent of cooking, but particularly since the development of agriculture, men have progressively been transforming their foods. Short of being *adapted* to these innovations, are we even sufficiently *adjusted* to them to be able to ingest them without ill effect?

"Man does not live by bread alone" is certainly true, but . . . *can he live by bread at all?* Upsetting as this may be, the answer seems to be, No.

Anopsotherapy is based on the discovery that when a human being eats any food *in its original state, its taste changes at some point from pleasant to unpleasant.* This means that when the organism has filled its need for that particular food, it no longer wants any more (even though it may still be hungry). However, this mechanism functions *only* with foods that have not been denatured in any way, and only when eaten in isolation, i.e., unmixed with others, unseasoned. The phenomenon does not occur with foods that have been frozen, cooked, chopped, ground, etc., or with extracts such as juices or oils. In nature, what an animal *wants* is one and the same as what it *needs.* Consequently, when dealing with foods whose structure evolved concurrently over millions of years with our own, our genetically determined senses of smell and taste should tell us not only *what* we need, but also *how much.* And indeed they do.

Obviously, the taste of a food is not to be found in the food, but in whoever is eating it. What a person needs (and therefore, what he perceives as attractive) depends on the overall molecular state of his body at that particular moment. For example, we seek water only when we're thirsty, and instinctively stop drinking when we've had enough. Could we not expect this to apply to food as well? With *original* food, it does. This is demonstrably true, and in a moment we will show you how you can prove it for yourself.

Cooking or otherwise modifying a food, however, alters its original molecular structure to which we are genetically adapted. Once cooked, it will taste the same *indefinitely* because its thermally modified structure will not trigger a taste-change response. As a consequence, we can continue to eat it with whatever satisfaction it provides until we're full, and ingest many times the amount we required. Furthermore, because our enzymes became adapted through evolution exclusively to the molecular structures of our native alimentary spectrum, they cannot correctly process the novel molecular structures produced by our culinary arts. Anyone who doubts that cooking alters the molecular structure of food, need only observe an egg-white in the frying pan as it becomes opaque.

Our organisms should perhaps, in theory, be able with no ill effects to eliminate substances eaten to excess, as well as the altered ones we are not adapted to and which are therefore toxic to us. But since we are rarely if ever eating foods that can be evaluated instinctively, we end up with enormous deficiencies of some needed nutrients, and toxic surplusses and accumulations of others. In a sense, we "make do" with modified foods, which we cannot metabolize properly but hold on to for lack of "the real thing." But this not-quite-rightness has disruptive effects at every level of our body's organization.

This would be mere speculation but for the observation that during early periods of practicing instinctive nutrition, and/or during the course of certain illnesses, waste materials from [Anopsological] eaters often carry the smell of cooked foods eaten years before in some cases. After a time, their feces, urine, and sweat become entirely odorless. During the course of certain illnesses, however, specific odors of cheese, cooked fruits, or mustard, will appear, showing that the illness is in effect detoxifying the body in a "useful" way. So it becomes necessary to think of certain microbes and viruses, *not* as "dangerous" pathogenic agents, but in a very different relationship. Once you have understood this point, you are unlikely to be too frightened by your symptoms if you fall ill. Furthermore, Instinctotherapy provides a method for treating or preventing most symptoms yourself.

This view departs from current medical philosophy with its emphasis on "war" against "dangerous invaders." It is based on observations of sickness and health exclusively in persons loaded from birth with accumulated residues from denatured nutrients, with no understanding of their effects or even of their existence. Its formulations reflect a metaphysics of the enemy without vs. the defenders within, reminiscent of the medieval concept of the Devil vs. the Lord. But life is not that simple.

Medicine, biochemistry, and genetics, are based on scientific analyses and abstractions produced by men, not by gods. We cannot know *everything* about *anything*. The human body is made up of some sixty thousand billion cells. They are of different types and sizes, but if we imagine a cell the size of a two-story house, a protein molecule would be like a beer can, an atom the size of a dust mote. Glucose passing through the intestinal mucous membrane does so at the rate of 100,000 billion molecules per second per square centimeter. The number of electro-colloidal processes occurring in an organism at any moment is beyond our comprehension, so we must simplify our understanding of them to suit the capacities of our intellects. We take note of some things and neglect the others, and postulate theories on the basis of what we've noticed and consider important. No crime here until we forget that nature contains more than we can see, and that the "laws" of nature are in fact made by man, since nature itself existed long before the evolutionary development of a neo-cortex capable of the notion of "laws" in the first place. Our life processes, however we may represent them, are infinitely more complex than our "intelligence" (and its representations) to which they give rise — whence the need for greater respect for nature *as given* than we usually show.

From the Anopsological viewpoint, diseases fall into two general categories: 1) those whose symptoms follow a predictable pattern, such as measles, diptheria, smallpox, and typhoid, and 2) those that follow no coherent sequence, which include cancers, multiple sclerosis, and psoriasis. Under Anopsological conditions, the symptoms of the program-type diseases are consistently so benign as to be practically undetectable. You will discover this yourself if you consistently eat this way. Where nutrition consists of genetically appropriate foods, a bout of flu will usually last for hours rather than days or weeks, and be associated with odors (usually "rotten" or cheese-like) that show its cleansing nature. This is true of most "diseases" whose symptoms follow predictable patterns and include odiferous discharges.

Their symptoms are often so very severe in people on "normal balanced diets" because of the huge accumulations of mismetabolized material produced by such diets, that need to be eliminated; and they are further amplified by denatured food ingested during the course of the illness, and by medicines intended to cure it. In many cases medicines do put an end to the symptoms, by suspending the [detoxification] process. But they preclude the system clean-out that would constitute a true cure.

We will discuss these "patterned illnesses" in greater depth in later chapters, and show how many chronic or acute conditions can be healed simply by eliminating from the diet the foods that caused the symptoms.

The second class of "diseases," in this frame of reference, are the ones that have no set pattern. They are also to a great extent a consequence of toxic accumulations the organism was *unable* to eliminate. It is generally known and readily admitted, for instance, that a number of insecticides, food preservatives and coloring agents, and synthetic sweeteners may produce cancers and/or other severe pathological conditions in laboratory animals, and should therefore not be used by humans. It has also been shown that many of these substances, antibiotics among them, will accumulate in animal and human tissues. It is apparent, however, that *any* substance which is too alien to be either fully used or discarded by the organism's biochemistry will accumulate and have some degree of pathological effect. Will the pathology disappear once the substance is removed? That is essentially what happens when instinctive nutrition is practiced correctly, unless the pathology has gone too far. Not only that, but it becomes apparent that so-called "normal" people or animals on a "normal balanced diet" should themselves be considered "abnormal" and deficient in comparison to people and animals whose nutrition is genetically correct.

If you decide to eat by instinct along the lines set forth in this book, you will probably be in for some pleasant surprises. Normally, if you do it correctly, within two or three days of beginning, any constipation, diarrhea, or digestive problems you had will have disappeared. Within four or five days, most pain will have subsided or disappeared completely, including inflammatory pain, arthritic pain, and migraine, with the exception of pain from physically damaged nerves (which may nevertheless be alleviated partially). This may seem unbelievable but it is so. Once they have eliminated the denatured-food toxins from their bodies, instinctively nourished people even become immune to the physical pain of a burn or a broken bone, except for a few seconds immediately following the event. If you eat this way consistently, you will prove it for yourself if you have an accident of this type.

You can expect nervous problems to quiet down dramatically after only a few days of instinctive eating, although you may experience transient crises as toxins are being eliminated from your body tissues via your bloodstream. But in a short time most nervousness and irritability will have subsided, and you will experience an improved *psycho*-physiological state, and increased ability to face problems with equanimity. This calming effect is particularly noticeable in animals, who have no knowledge that such a thing "should" happen. Anopsologically fed pigs have straight, not corkscrew-like tails, and tend to wag them like dogs. Cats fed original foods do not startle or chase insects, and will not bare their claws even when picked up by the tail.

You stand to become much healthier than the average "healthy" person. You can expect to feel more energetic on less sleep. You can expect to lose your excess fat, and you will feel no need to drink or smoke. If you practice instinctive nutrition correctly, you will not be subject to hypoglycemic mood swings. You will become immune to infections in cuts or burns, whose healing time will be about half what is "normal." You will be immune to catching colds, and will be able to stand cold weather without great discomfort or ill effect.

Women who have been eating this way for a time can expect to experience little or no pain when giving birth, and labor is likely to be a matter of minutes rather than hours. Furthermore, the waters will break at the *end* of the process rather than at the beginning, so that the baby is propelled hydraulically through the birth canal. This phenomenon has been observed many times in instinctively fed women, and is presumably what nature intended, that unnatural nutrition prevents.

Anopsotherapy has been applied successfully in cases of severe pathology including cataracts, herpes, colitis, psoriasis, alcoholism, asthma, allergies, diabetes, staphyloccocal infections and ulcers. It has saved the lives of cancer and leukemia patients, ended tremor and paralysis in persons with multiple sclerosis, eliminated pain in patients with arthritis and glaucoma. A number of case histories and reports are included in later chapters, and provide an indication of what genetically proper nutrition can do.

Because Anopsotherapy is so broadly effective, it sounds *too good to be true* — so that you may feel it is not. But if it *is* true . . . then why didn't anybody discover it before?

One answer to this question is: *tradition*. No culture exists on earth at this time — nor has any existed for many thousands of years — that does not mix, season, cook or otherwise denature its foods. Cooking, in particular, is everywhere assumed to be not only natural, but necessary. Research in medicine and nutrition has rarely if ever questioned this premise, so that the discovery that we possess a nutritional instinct, that only functions normally with foods in their original, unmodified state, was necessarily a long time in coming.

Chapter 2

The Instinctive Message

Part I

> Instinct: "A natural impulse or propensity that incites animals, including man, to the actions that are essential to their existence, preservation and development . . . a propensity prior to experience and independent of instruction."

"Instincts" for various reasons are not in vogue at this time. Many consider them to be "base," or vile . . . or worse. Others deny their existence. Sigmund Freud, who postulated an unpopular "Death Instinct," no doubt had something to do with it. We currently prefer other explanations for *why* we do *what* we do. We prefer to say we have "needs" that require fulfilling, or in this computer age, speak about having been "programmed," genetically, socially or otherwise to act in one way or another. But instinct is for the birds, the bees and the beavers — not for us. (It is understood that we are phylogenetically descended from fish and monkeys, for whom it is legitimate to have instincts, since they do not have languages, science or "understanding" such as we do.) But it is generally assumed that if instinct does in fact exist in humans, it is so weak as to be negligible.

Is this true, however? Because of our genetic heritage, human beings are in many ways similar to animals, particularly the higher vertebrates. New-born babies particularly resemble animals in their behaviors. Until they grow a cerebral cortex enabling them to generate higher-order representations, they act on feelings (or "senses", or "instinct") alone. No rules, no principles, or recipes guide them until they grow older. The higher brain functions, once they develop, may repress or deviate the earlier ones, but do not eliminate them. So the "animal-like" behaviors of the infant remain present — if in check — in the adult.

One of the very first things a new-born baby wants to do is eat. Under natural circumstances, he cries out his want, and the mother responds by offering her breast. This behavior can be observed in cats, pigs, horses and every other mammal. And almost without exception in the animal world, mother is able (and willing) to provide enough milk for baby's wants as long as he needs it.

Under normal circumstances in the human world, however, mother is frequently unable or unwilling to breast-feed baby. In these cases, baby will usually be fed a solution of modified cow's milk. There may be nothing wrong with this. But it should be noted that in the animal world, no piglet has ever been observed to suckle a goat, no kitten a dog, no mouse a rabbit, no weasel a fox. No human baby has ever been seen to suckle a cow, either.

Within hours of birth, human babies are able and happy to eat fresh mango, banana, papaya and a variety of other foods that the mother either pre-masticates or gives them whole to suck upon. They will, in fact, frequently abandon the breast and clamor for fruit the mother is eating (and whose smell has reached them) while nursing.

Let us ask: How does this come about? How does an animal — or a human baby — know what it needs to eat? To put it another way, does an animal or baby "know" what it needs at all? Is it a case of "mama knows best"?

As far as animals, at least, are concerned, a seemingly obvious answer would be, "The animal doesn't really 'know' what's good for it — it just eats whatever is appealing, whatever has an attractive smell and taste." Let's explore this and do an experiment. It will probably be most easily understood if we use a dog. You need not take our word as to the outcome, since you can easily repeat it yourself. If you don't own a dog you can possibly borrow one.

For this experiment, we will not fill Fido's bowl with dog biscuits, canned dog food or any other mixture or commercial product. We will offer him a banana. Dogs sometimes like bananas, and this *"sometimes"* is very, very important. If Fido isn't in the mood for banana *at this time*, he'll turn away from it, and we'll have to try again later. But we might also try giving him a raw carrot, or fresh strawberries, or some other fresh fruit or vegetable.

There is a fair chance, however, that Fido will go for the banana. We're going to feed it to him bite by bite. If he finishes the first banana, we'll give him another one, and keep going as long as he's taking it. For at some point, he'll take no more. He'll turn away, he'll disdain our offering. This is exactly what baby will do when mother offers him some food he doesn't want. But Fido is more fortunate than baby, because no one ever declared that bananas were "good for dogs" — whereas bananas, by tradition if not by prescription, are "good for babies."

Once Fido has stopped responding to the banana offerings, we may assume that he's not hungry anymore. But let's test this hypothesis, and offer him a piece of raw meat. Does he go for it? If he does, then he was still hungry, only he was no longer hungry *for banana*.

This may seem self-evident or pointless. So he's no longer hungry for banana — so what?

This "so what?" is one of the most fundamental questions nutritional science has ever neglected to ask. But in order to understand why, you should undertake an experiment on yourself. You should do more than simply read about it. *Doing* this simple experiment will enable you to grasp a fundamental truth, if ever there was one, from within your experience. "Intellectual" understanding alone will not suffice. It is a truth that every one of us knew at birth, and repressed from the time we were first given food we didn't want or need, but had no means to refuse. If you do not actually do this experiment, you may tend to dismiss what follows as nonsense. You can prove for yourself that it isn't.

This is a tasting experiment and easy to do. You may use bananas, pineapples, or any other fresh fruit that has not been denatured. This point is extremely important. Fruit must be used that has not been frozen, ground, cooked, treated or otherwise modified in any way. It must be fruit in its original state, the way it was when it came off the tree, or bush or whatever it was it grew on. And it must not be mixed with anything else — not with other fruit in a salad, not with sugar.

This experiment will also work with honey, vegetables, fish and other foods. But it will not work with any food that is not in its original state, and since so much processing goes on that may not be evident, we are suggesting it be done exclusively with fresh original fruit that can readily be recognized as such.

Choose the fruit you will use by smelling it. If it smells good, it will probably taste good. Take the apples or pears or pineapples or melons or whatever you bought, and settle down where you won't be disturbed. Eat slowly, and pay close attention to the taste. If you don't like the taste from the first bite, try some other fruit — or wait a day or two until that particular fruit tastes good from the outset.

As you eat your way through the fruit, there will come a point where *the taste changes*. Assuming it was pleasant at first, it will progressively become unpleasant, and if you persist, it will become unbearable. For instance, a pineapple that you found sweet and delicious at the outset, will at some point become so biting that you will be unable to eat any more. An apple, initially delectable, will at some point become raspy, woolly, and so unpleasant that you are unable to swallow it.

This is the instinctive, alliesthetic Taste Barrier. It is a biochemical reaction of the organism. Every one of us once knew about it, because when we were babies it was our guide for what we wanted, which is one and the same thing as what we needed. It is how every living animal of every species knows, without recourse to dietetic theory, precisely what it needs to eat, and how much. It is an organismic message that says, unequivocally, when something good-tasting turns into something bad-tasting: I have had all I need.

This is the way every species of living organism "knows" what it needs to survive. It eats what smells or tastes good, and turns away from what smells or tastes bad. When it has fulfilled its need for one particular food, it has also fulfilled its want, and turns away. This is what Fido did; and what you did too, if you carried out the experiment.

The human senses of smell and taste would provide an infallible guide as to what types and amounts of food our organisms require, but for one thing: human "intelligence." Human beings are the only living species to feed on the milk of another species, to cultivate grains and other plant types, and to mix, season, ferment, and above all, cook their foods. But the alliesthetic taste change does not occur with any food that is not in its original state. This unfortunate and demonstrable truth has profound implications for the well-being of every human being on earth.

> . . . it is important to keep in mind that, in general, animal life has largely escaped many of the degenerative processes which affect modern white peoples. We ascribe this to animal instinct in the matter of food selection. It is possible that man has lost through disuse some of the normal faculty for consciously recognizing body requirements. In other words, the only hunger of which we now are conscious is a hunger for energy to keep us warm and to sup-

ply power. In general, we stop eating when an adequate amount of energy has been provided, whether or not the body building and repairing materials have been included in the food.'

Part II

Almost any normal person should have little difficulty successfully carrying out the taste-change experiment outlined above. If you did it, you may have noticed that upon returning immediately to an original food whose taste has turned bad, its smell will have become unattractive as well.

If you have eaten your fill and are no longer hungry, you may even notice that you can find no food smells at all that attract you. And if you are to experiment further, you will find that *non-food* smells remain unaffected. The perfume you liked before eating will seem just as appealing afterward. Why is this so?

This is so because human beings have built-in mechanisms that developed through evolution with respect to the smells that would ensure their well-being, but not with incidental ones. For any animal in nature, needed foods *must* smell good as long as they are needed, and unneeded or poisonous foods *must* smell unattractive if that animal is to survive. It would also be imperative that danger smells and sexual smells trigger the proper reactions for a species to thrive. But there would be no reason for mechanisms to evolve with respect to smells that were irrelevant to survival.

An experiment was carried out by a physiology research group in Lyon, France to explore how odors varied before and after eating.² Two groups of volunteers were first asked to rate the pleasantness/unpleasantness of 10 different substances on a scale of −2 (very unattractive) to 0 (neutral) to +2 (very attractive). Three groups of test items were used: 1) *food odors:* meat, cheese, fish and honey; 2) *odors from non-foods frequently associated with foods:* tobacco, wine and coffee; and 3) *non-food odors:* lavender, sodium hypochlorite and India Ink.

After rating the odors, one group had a meal of bread, butter, ham, french-fries, concentrated sweet milk and an orange. The control group simply didn't eat. After the meal, both groups were asked to smell and rate each sample seven times at 20 minute intervals.

The before and after ratings of the food odors were markedly different. Before eating, the food odors were almost universally attractive to both groups (with some variation in the degree of attractiveness partly as a result of personal preferences and/or individual criteria for grading them). But however attractive a food odor may have been before the meal, its rating after the meal was significantly lower — while the control group (the ones that hadn't eaten) continued to find them attractive.

However, the meal, or lack of it, had no significant effect on the ratings of non-food odors. Tobacco, coffee, wine, lavender, sodium hypochlorite and ink smelled just as pleasant or unpleasant to the eaters after the meal as they had before, and did not vary for the control group either.

The researchers concluded that we possess an *alliesthetic* (meaning: a change in sensory experience) mechanism that makes food relatively attractive when we need it and unattractive when we don't — and that this is an innate phenomenon since it functions with foods, but not with artificial odors from non-foods. It is unfortunate that no distinction was made by the experimenters between *original* food and denatured food, for the before-and-after differences would have been even more pronounced — a contention you can verify for yourself.

There is' one necessary inference the researchers did not explicitly draw from the results of the experiment, possibly because it seemed obvious: *the attractiveness or repulsiveness we experience when smelling a food depends on our body's biochemical state.* We will not be attracted to a smell when our chemistry has "shut the door" on it.

If we *are* attracted to food when we *don't* need it, then something must have gone wrong with our internal control and sensing systems. If we *are not* attracted to food when we *do* need it, something must also be wrong. And it is easy to see what it is: Millions of years of evolutionary development did not prepare our bodies or our built-in alimentary sensing systems (our instinct) to cope with denatured foods, which simply did not exist until recently. Since we cannot evaluate them correctly by instinct, we become overloaded with some nutrients and deficient in others – overfed and undernourished, as it were – and as a result, our attraction/revulsion system is confused.

You will discover after eating by instinct for a time, that smells and tastes become clearer than ever before, and a clear-cut alliesthetic response with original foods will become as spontaneous and natural as experiencing hot and cold. In fact, you will learn to recognize when a supposedly original food is not in its original state – because its taste doesn't change.

[1] Weston A. Price, *Nutrition and Physical Degeneration,* The Price-Pottenger Nutrition Foundation, San Diego, 1970.
[2] *Effects of Eating a Meal on the Pleasantness of Food and Non-food Odors in Man* by Duclaux, Feisthauer & Cabanac, *Physiology and Behavior,* Vol. 10, 1973.

Chapter 3

The Instinctively Balanced Diet

It is unlikely that anyone even slightly informed in matters of nutrition would dispute the following statements. Yet they contain a fundamental error. Can you spot it?

> The list of raw materials we need from our environment is a long one, and the list is largely what nutrition is all about. We need calcium ions, phosphorous ions, sodium ions, potassium ions, chloride ions, magnesium ions, ferric or ferrous ions, zinc ions, manganese ions, copper ions, cobalt ions, molybdenum ions, iodine, leucine, isoleucine, valine, methionine, theonine, phenylalanine, some form of Vitamin A, some form of Vitamin D, some form of Vitamin E, some form of Vitamin K, Vitamin C, thiamine, riboflavin, pantothenate, niacinamide, biotin, folic acid, pyridoxine, and Vitamin B_{12}.

Unbelievable as it may seem, we need all of these elements in about the right amounts every day (or every two days) or we suffer. Furthermore, there is excellent evidence that all of the elements listed constitute absolute needs. If we fail to get them and run out of our reserves, we will surely die. It gives one an odd feeling to realize that our very existence depends every day on the practical solution of an equation with 40 or more variables.[1]

Did you spot it — the *"Minimum Daily Requirement"* concept? It is to be found on labels on vitamin bottles, cereal boxes, bread packages. It underlies the precept of the daily apple or the morning dose of orange juice. Were it true, the human race would not have survived long enough to become human. There were no supermarkets in the jungle; such calculated balancing acts would have been impossible.

We do not have a "Minimum Daily Requirement" for sex, and we do not have one for food, either. A minimal amount of the named nutrients, along with others, must be present in the organism if it is not to suffer from malnutrition. But the minimum amount of nutrients essential for health is not an *average* of the minimum amount that might be required over the course of several months or a year.

This becomes dramatically clear from observations of Instinctotherapy patients eating their way to health. Their requirement for some particular nutrients (and others) on any given day, or over a given period, may be so massive as to preclude all others — but once it has been filled, it may not again make itself felt for many weeks. Nor are nutritional requirements ever the same for two different people on any given day, or for a given individual on succeeding days.

A simple analogy will make it clear why this is so.

Let us say we are going to build (or rebuild) not a body, but a house. So we are going to use . . . not proteins, vitamins, amino acids, glucose, etc., but cement, rafters, wiring, pipes, window panes, shingles and so on. Let's say it's a 100-day project. Now it's mealtime (supply time) on the building site and here comes the lunch wagon (delivery truck). It is scheduled to come every day for 100 days, and if it is to provide a "balanced diet" (of materials), then naturally, on the first and every succeeding day it will be carrying: 1/100th of the cement requirement, 1% of the rafters, 1% of the wiring, etc. Shall we start building? How can we?

How can we build when at each stage of construction we need *all* the material required at that stage? At the outset we will need cement and reinforcing rods for the foundations – and window panes not at all. Many items not only can wait, but *must.*(Things have to proceed in a particular order or chaos will ensue.)

When the body needs supplies for whatever it's building (or rebuilding) at a particular time, it needs the *full amount* of the requirement or it must leave the job unfinished. But just exactly what it does need, and when and how much, can only be determined by the individual himself, never by prescription. And it can be correctly determined only by obedience to the body's sensory (instinctive) cues with native foods, the greater the variety to choose from the better. Because with these foods, we can only want what we need, and when we have had all we need, we will want no more.

This is not speculation. Instinct may lead a person to eat as many as forty or fifty raw egg yolks at a sitting before the taste becomes unpleasant or before he feels full – and then to again eat practically nothing but raw egg yolks at the next meal, and the next, possibly for days or weeks on end. And then, abruptly, eggs will hold no more attraction, and the person will find himself making full meals of oranges and pineapples, or oysters, or spinach.

Why is this so?

The reason, obviously, is that there was a tremendous deficiency in some area that was demanding priority. And once it was fulfilled, but not before, other requirements could make themselves felt.

It is true, as stated above, that unless a minimal amount of each and every nutrient our body requires is present, we will suffer from malnutrition. But the implication that there is a static, fixed minimum for human beings in general, is wrong. Particularly in a therapeutic context, the minimum we require may greatly exceed any theoretical determination. And conversely, the ingestion of a supposedly "necessary" nutrient may be toxic because it exceeds the body's requirement for it at that particular moment. Give orange juice (that provides no alliesthetic cues) to an instinctive eater, and the excess may well give him a headache or a rash (and it will produce ill effects in "normal" eaters as well, even if they are unable to recognize them).

The notion of a "balanced" diet is a trap for many beginning practitioners of instinctive nutrition. Someone who has not been attracted to beef, for example, for two or three weeks, may tell himself, "I haven't had any beef for so long — I'm sure I need some," and proceed to eat steaks in which he takes little if any pleasure and that leave him feeling unwell.

For an individual to be truly well fed, his diet must be properly *un*balanced. But only his instinct, not prescriptions, can lead him to eat what he really needs and tell him when to stop.

Since this instinct — our genetic alimentary programming — works only with the foods it is familiar with from eons of natural cohabitation, let us now see which ones these might be.

---

[1] Quoted by Schultz & Myers in *Metabolic Aspects of Health*, Discovery Press, Kentfield, 1979.

Chapter 4

What is a "Natural" Food?

The word "natural" has been perverted. Everyone knows what it means — and it means something different to practically everyone. Countless "natural" products are on the market, even in vending machines. Some are said to be more natural than others. So-called "biological" produce, for example, is thought to be more natural than foods grown with chemical fertilizers. It is also widely believed that "natural" = "good for you". Let us wonder about this.

First of all: what food is "natural" for mankind as a species? Are we "naturally" (i.e., innately) carnivorous, ichthyvorous, omni-vorous, fructivorous, vegetarian or something else? There are numerous schools of thought on this subject, some of them of a religious nature, others philosophical, yet others claiming to be founded on scientific enquiry. There is generally little agreement among them.

For another thing: what food is "natural" for a given individual at a given time? Should he eat fish at least once a week, have orange juice every day, avoid chocolate, eat plenty of fibers? Should he consume only fruit that is in season? Are sugars alright when it's cold outside, harmful when it's not? Should a person with the flu consume citrus fruits? Should a pregnant woman eat a lot of cheese? Should foods be mixed together in one way but not in another? Countless theories exist in this area as well, in endless contradiction.

For the most part, answers to both these types of questions are provided by the culture we live in. Recipes, including remedies for the upsets they may produce, are passed on from mother to daughter. The former as "secrets," the latter as "wisdom." Every society has its popular nutritional traditions, habits, maxims, biases, and taboos. Culinary folklore is so pervasive that it affects even "scientific" nutritional maxims and practices. Here, the physician will eschew soft-boiled eggs for his patient because they are "hard to digest." There, he will prescribe them because "nothing is easier to digest." As we will see, however, both theories are wrong.

Different countries thrive on different foods. Americans eat vast amounts of meat, wheat and dairy products. Beans and corn are the staples in Mexico, rice and vegetables in China, potatoes in Germany, cabbage and herring in Russia and so forth. Fortunately, the inhabitants of these countries do not limit themselves exclusively to these diets, but generally, they consider them to be "basic." And they assume that these staples are "natural" for the species Homo Sapiens to which they belong.

It must be emphasized that the nutritional habits of any culture are indeed precisely that — *habits*. They came into being the same way the language, music, and art of that culture arose: by circumstance and by chance. They are not necessarily "natural," i.e., *native* to men the way plankton is native to whales.

It could be argued that since man is a "natural" phenomenon on earth, any artifice he produces is "natural" as well, and that the T.V. commercials made by men are as natural in the scheme of the universe as the dams made by beavers. The argument carries some weight, since it is indeed "natural" for men to be "unnatural," to live by the rules and assumptions of an arbitrary man-made cultural system, and to create things not found in nature. In order to avoid confusion, therefore, let us define "natural" as analogous to "primal", "unaffected by the human cerebral cortex."

This point is fundamental, because for many millions of years of his evolutionary development, man and his predecessors did not possess, or at any rate did not use, enough cerebral cortex to affect much of anything. He lived in an environment he could not transform. He might find a cave to live in, but he couldn't build one. He could eat a fish found dead on the beach, but he couldn't catch it in the ocean. He was dependent upon whatever his surroundings provided, the way it provided it. He was also *adapted* to the foods in his environment. Had he not been, he would not have survived as a species until the time came when fire was mastered, the stone axe invented, or the discovery made that seeds could be planted in the earth.

What were men eating in those days so incredibly distant, before they developed higher-brain structures enabling them to invent ways to transform their environment and their food? By exploring this question, perhaps we can determine what foods are truly natural for humans. Obviously, we cannot go back and observe them first-hand. But we can determine them in part by exclusion, by asking: what foods are *unnatural* for humans? What were our distant forebears *not* eating? This should give us a pretty good start.

For one thing, they were not drinking milk. Cows had not been domesticated, and a wild cow would hardly have stood still long enough to be milked. Even assuming they were interested in doing it, and that someone had figured out how, they would have needed a vessel to hold the milk. They had not yet invented such a thing.

We might imagine a group of distant prehistoric men surrounding a wild cow, and taking turns suckling her teats. But it seems unlikely. For one thing, looking around us in nature, we find no case of one species of mammal ingesting the milk of another. We do not see squirrels suckling goats or weasels suckling foxes. And in no case do we find an adult member of a species ingesting milk at all — only the children. So we can infer that even same-species milk is unnatural for adults.

Is non-human milk natural for humans? Many human babies have "allergic" reactions to it, sometimes fatal. Most babies cease to have such reactions after a short time, and are said to have accomodated to it. Their reactions are not perceived as an organic protest, which is what they are. On the contrary, mothers and pediatricians are happy when baby has learned to tolerate milk. That way he can be given what's "good for him." Thanks to our technological ingenuity, it is now possible to remove the lactose from milk, so intolerant babies (and adults) can drink it. Why is it so important to be able to do this? Well — because we *believe* it is.

Our culture holds that milk is a "natural" food, and that babies and children need calcium from it to grow strong bones and teeth. From their fossil remains, we know that our prehistoric ancestors had strong bones and teeth without it. It seems probable that their bones were somewhat less brittle than ours, and fractured less readily. Whatever the case, if the early humans had truly needed non-human milk to survive, they would not have.

Another thing our predecessors were not eating is rice. They might have stumbled on a growth of wild rice, and explored the taste of its grains. The might even have liked it, but that seems doubtful. Human beings today do not generally care for, or manage to eat, uncooked rice — although many birds and rodents enjoy it. Furthermore, rice would have been scarce. It was only eight to ten thousand years ago that man began to cultivate cereals. Over the millions of years preceding agriculture, it seems unlikely that rice would have been plentiful enough to provide much food.

In fact, it seems improbable that *any* cereal would have been on our ancestral menu. Wild wheat, barley, corn or oats might have been of occasional passing interest. But without methods of cultivating and threshing them in quantity, they could have provided only a very small part of pre-humankind's nutrition. Even assuming an abundance of one or another of these grains, the problem of threshing them a handful at a time would not have made them popular.

We must remember that until they developed some rudimentary technology and civilization, our ancestors chose their food the way animals do, the way our cousins the monkeys do. They ate what smelled and tasted good, and avoided whatever was unpleasant to their senses. They had no other guide. Thanks to the automatic mechanisms of their biochemistry, what they *needed* was what they *wanted*. How, then, did we become so divorced from our alimentary instinct that we need to rely on laboratory analyses to know what is "good for us"?

The answer to this question lies in our inability to correctly evaluate any food that is not in the native, original state it was in over the hundreds of millions of years during which our biochemistry was evolving adaptively with it. With original foods, when our organism has had its fill, the taste becomes unpleasant. This does not happen with denatured food whose molecular structure is alien to our biochemical programming. The modified molecular structure of such food will not trigger our alliesthetic (taste-change) response. Once a food has been denatured − by cooking, for instance − its taste will remain unchanged for as long as we care to eat it.

Once humans discovered how fire could be used for cooking, they were on a one-way trip to metabolic chaos and organic disharmony. They had tied a knot they couldn't undo, that we, their descendants, have rendered practically inextricable.

In order to understand this, let us imagine a tribe of Homo Erectus somewhere in the forest, say around 400,000 B.C. They are gathered near a fire, eating yams and other foods collected earlier in the day. The ones who are eating yams are those whose bodies need nutrients the yams contain: this is what makes them smell and taste good. Those who do not need yams are not attracted to them.

Whatever they're eating, they are eating it raw, the way it came off a tree or out of the ground. It has never occurred to any of them to mix, grind, pound, heat or do anything else to an attractive piece of food other than eat it.

One member of the group, call him Onemug¹, has eaten less than a fourth of a yam when the taste becomes unattractive. Carelessly he throws it down, and it rolls onto the edge of the fire, unnoticed. And there, it begins to bake. And it begins to smell. And the smell is stronger than ever a yam smelled before. The smell reaches Onemug's nose, and it is good. So Onemug follows his nose, and takes up the baked yam and begins to eat it. He can do so now, because the taste has become good again. So Onemug eats the rest of the yam. The yam's molecular structure, modified by heat, no longer causes its taste to change from good to bad.

A day or so later, Onemug is hungry, but all the tribe has found to eat that day is yams. Thanks to the cooking, Onemug had been able to eat more yam than he actually needed, so his organism is still overloaded with it. As a result, naturally, he finds raw yam unattractive. But Onemug is a genius: he remembers that the hot yam from the fire was good: he associates: fire + yam = good. On an impulse, he pushes a yam into the fire. And sure enough, after a while an attractive smell comes to his nose. And he is able to eat the yam with a degree of pleasure until he's full.

Of course, the other members of the tribe smell the cooked yam too, and begin to follow suit. So all of them begin to eat yams, not until the body has had its fill of the nutrients yams contain, but until the belly has room for no more. And naturally, the next day, because they don't need them, none of them is attracted to raw yams any longer.

This brings upon the tribe an unexpected change in the way it lives. Up to now, yams in their natural state were delicious. Now, however, they have to be cooked or they can't be eaten.

Instinct has to be tricked or it will stop the organism from overloading itself with substances it doesn't need.

Thus is birth given to the artifice of cooking. It is not yet an "art" in the sense of *haute cuisine* but it must inevitably become one. For by disrupting the dynamic structure of a food, cooking kills its taste: each mouthful tastes just like the last. Since it will not trigger an alliesthetic response, it will not become unpalatable. But it *will* be boring, because the taste of cooked food does not vary.

Over the centuries, ways will be found to "enliven" it, to make it interesting and pleasurable to eat. Food in its original state will of itself be more pleasurable than any artifice can ever make it, but only if the body needs it. However, once the organism has become saturated with remnants of denatured food (which it can neither use or eliminate because biochemically it "doesn't know how"), then the senses of smell and taste themselves become denatured, and dulled. Thus must leaves, herbs, spices, ferments, oils, extracts, mixing, baking, roasting, basting and boiling, etc., be called upon to provide some flavor where none remains. The relationship between the dynamic molecular effects of these procedures on the food, and the effects of the food on the human organism, have only recently become a subject for scientific enquiry – which has generally assumed along with everyone else, that cooking is perfectly "natural" for humans.*

Is bread "natural"? What about salads? What about apple pie, mushroom soup, roast beef, French-fried potatoes?

Prehistoric archeological remains indicate that meat from hunted animals has been on the human menu for a long, long time. Studies of monkeys have shown that these close genetic cousins of ours also occasionally eat meat – uncooked. The Anopsological study of new-born babies shows that infants may spontaneously reach for raw beef and other meats whose smells

---

* Some people ask *why* cooked food tastes better to them than raw food. Why does a woman with makeup and a bikini seem more exciting than simply when naked? Cooking is an *art*, closely linked to cultural tastes. Once you become nutritionally balanced by instinct, cooking doesn't appeal like it did before.

are attractive, beginning shortly after birth. Children and adults of all ages regularly find that raw, naturally raised beef, rabbit, pork, chicken, or goat, can be gloriously delicious on occasion, with the taste-change occurring after varying amounts have been consumed.

They may also report nervousness, physical pain and other more severe symptoms when they have eaten meat from an animal that was itself fed unnatural food.

We need to explore this scene-behind-the-scene in trying to determine what food is "natural" for humans. Any organism "is" what it eats. Feed a pig garbage and his meat will taste of garbage. Feed him carrots, apples, or peas, and his meat will be sweet. Crayfish raised in muck will taste of muck, and humans fed junk will smell – and taste – of it. There is no need to eat your neighbor to verify this contention; one need only taste his blood on the occasion of cutting himself. Instinctively fed people will carry almost no taste at all. It should also be noted in passing that the menstrual blood from instinctively fed women is also practically without taste or odor (and there is very little of it).

Is wheat a natural food for cattle? What were cattle eating before men had put ropes around their necks? Can we imagine a wild steer being attracted to a growth of wild wheat, and spontaneously eating the grains? The wheat was not threshed, and growing wheat husks are spiked – could this have been a native food for wild cattle through the ages?

Cattle are fed grains in order to put fat on them. If someone is selling a product by the pound, the more pounds he sells the more he makes. In our society, this is allowable. In fact, in America (and in many other places) we value "more" of many things, and for most of us "bigger" = "better". Mother is proud that baby is big. The gardener is proud of his big tomatoes. We want to raise neither small children, small fruit nor small cattle. So we feed our children, produce and beasts whatever will increase their volume and weight.

Cows do not get fat on grass — only on grains, or in more general terms, only on foods to which their biochemistry is not genetically adapted. This applies to any animal, and it applies to humans. Humans get fat on bread, cooked sugars, cooked potatoes, milk, cheese and practically any other denatured food their bodies can only process in part, but have learned to tolerate.

Abnormal food can only be used in part, and eliminated in part, because it is alien to our built-in biochemical programming — so what happens to whatever has not been processed? Not used, and not discarded, it remains. And over time, more and more remains. It remains in the cells and between the cells and denatures their relationships with one another and within themselves. And it takes up space and creates electro-static bonds to hold ions in place that would normally move elsewhere, so there is too much of this here and too little of that there.

The pseudo-metabolism of unnatural nutrients is not the topic of this discussion, but these remarks will, I hope, serve to emphasize a simple truth: if whatever we are eating was itself not eating whatever was natural *for it*, then we in turn will be ingesting whatever it still contains that it was unable to fully use or eliminate. Feeding occurs in self-reflexive cycles: our food fed on food that in turn fed on food, indefinitely.

The dangers of man-made toxins such as mercury in fish or pesticides on fruit, are widely recognized. The dangers of man-made toxins in the form of grain-only for chickens, oats for horses, wheat for cattle are not. These may be "natural" foods in that they are products of nature (although probably denatured by artificial selection) but unless they were part of the eater's native alimentary spectrum, they are *unnatural* for him, and will produce unnatural effects in him, and subsequently, in whatever feeds upon him.

But let us move on. Is orange juice — freshly squeezed orange juice, not concentrated or frozen — is that, at least, "natural"?

Orange juice may contain some molecular structures the body needs, but it does *not* contain some that have never been reported upon by our analytical laboratories, but which are to be found *only* in an orange as-a-whole: the whatever-it-is that causes the taste of a whole orange to become biting and/or acid at some point, so that the eater is forced to stop when he has had enough. For orange juice, even freshly squeezed, can be drunk to excess, and the overdose will be toxic. It can bring about headaches, stomach cramps, "allergic" reactions — any number of mild or more severe symptoms of poisoning. This will never happen with whole oranges.

Foods in their original state cannot poison us. Denatured ones can. If raw mushrooms smell good and taste good, they will not harm us. If while eating them the taste becomes disagreeable, this organic statement that we have had enough will automatically stop us. Denatured mushrooms, on the other hand, can be deadly. Many studies have been published on the types of mushrooms we can cook and still eat (with seasoning to make them interesting) without harm. But no one knows *how many* cooked mushrooms of any given type we can eat, because that will vary from one person to the next, and from day to day. Instinct provides an automatic answer.

It is for these same reasons that soft-boiled eggs may be "hard to digest" or "easy to digest." Depending on the state of the organism, one or two or three dozen raw eggs at one sitting may have no ill effect — or even one raw egg might produce an upset stomach. Once they are cooked (and particularly once salt or pepper has been added) we cannot predict what will happen. With an undenatured egg, we know the instant it touches our tongue.

There is an important difference between "natural" raw foods eaten separately, and "natural" *mixed* raw foods. When two or more foods are mixed together, smell and taste become confused. Our senses will tell us immediately whether a tomato or an onion is a needed (and therefore attractive) item. But if we cut them up and eat them together we can no longer know. We cannot properly evaluate more than one smell or taste at a time. It is currently believed that salads are "natural" and "healthy." It is certainly possible. Taking turnips, cucumbers, radishes, endives, lettuce and other vegetables separately, we will know which ones our body needs. Once we have tossed them with salt, pepper, oil, vinegar or the complex chemical compounds sold in strangely shaped bottles bearing exotic names, we will not.

Frozen food also creates a problem. When water freezes within the cells of a food, it expands and among other things, breaks down the cellular membranes. So-called "fresh frozen" fruits and vegetables may have been fresh before they were frozen — but they certainly no longer are when they're thawed. Most will have lost a good part of their smell and taste. More importantly, our alliesthetic mechanisms do not function with them: freshly thawed (but uncooked) foods will not trigger a change of taste when the organism has reached a point of no-more-need. In theory at least, frozen foods will generally be less denatured than canned ones. But they are not "natural" in the Anopsological sense.

The food we most often eat with all the ones mentioned above, and others, is *bread*. Seemingly endless varieties of bread are on the market, containing or not containing whatever the consumer is presumed to desire or fear, many of their labels claiming "only natural ingredients." If the hybrid corn that grew in a field may be said to be "natural," the oil extracted from it cannot. The cane was certainly "natural," but the sugar refined from its juices is not. If the flour came from a calculatingly bred strain of wheat that is drought resistant (or unattractive to some form of bacteria or fungus) than it contains special substances that will also have unique peculiarities within the human intestinal tract.

If wheat (or corn or rye) was not part of man's original alimentary spectrum when raw, it is even less so when cooked. The more complex its structure, the more complex will the molecular alterations be when its temperature is raised during baking. This is to say that the closer the wheat is to its "natural" state (i.e., "whole"), the more complex will the chemical compounds be that are created during baking, and the more difficult will it be for the human organism to process them. Whole-wheat bread must necessarily be more disruptive to the metabolism than white bread. And this is, in fact, how it is experienced by instinctive eaters who have experimented with it.

Bread in any shape or form is not a "natural" food for human beings. Unleavened bread, containing only flour and water, already makes use of an unnatural food for humans, which it chemically compounds at high temperature. When added to this we find sugar and yeast and the gasses these produce, plus oils, salts, extracts, and even synthetic vitamins and mineral complements — what do we have?

The answer is: *we don't know.* The human organism possesses only a limited number of enzymes with which to process its food — enzymes that it developed over millions of years of evolution. When presented with bread, among other cooked and denatured foods, it does "not know" what it has to deal with. Its metabolism is in disarray — confused. And the submicroscopic disorder to which it is subjected becomes microscopic disorder, which becomes macroscopic disorder called anemia, obesity, arthritis, hepatitis, allergy, heart disease, gallstones, hypoglycemia, impotence, "nervous tension" . . .

Man, we are told, cannot live by bread alone. We might somewhat more accurately say he cannot live by bread at all — or by any other food for which his genetic code is not prepared.

> *The foods we eat are usually divided into four basic groups: meat and fish, vegetables and fruit, milk and milk products, and breads and cereals. Two or more daily servings from each are now considered necessary for a balanced diet, but adults living before the development of agriculture and animal husbandry derived all their nutrients from the first two food groups: they apparently consumed cereal grains rarely if at all, and they had no dairy foods whatsoever.*
>
> *(From Paleolithic Nutrition by S. B. Eaton and M. Kowner in The New England Journal of Medicine, Jan., 1985.)*

' *In German-speaking Switzerland, one = "ein" and mug = "stein".*

Chapter 5

Some Effects of Unnatural Foods

Of course, we are *humans*, not animals. "Animals" are just not quite like humans, obviously.

But "not quite" also means "almost." By denying that humans are almost like animals we can guiltlessly remain blind to their pain while killing them for "sport," imprisoning them for profit or using and abusing them for "science." We can do this because we are "higher" than they are. Higher than the highest.

But not quite. Relative to our weight, we have bigger brains than other animals, and thanks to our cerebral cortices, we possess the unique capacity to represent with symbols, objects and situations that are not physically present — and which may not even exist at all. Thanks to this capacity, we can create things not found in nature, and produce so many of them that we even forget we are part of nature at all.

But part of nature we are. We are still subject to the "laws of life," whatever they may be, and our "animal nature" determines our behaviors today as much as it did when we lived in the jungle. However warped or buried it may have become by the rituals and values of our culture, our animal status still is nearly intact.

A lot of thought has gone into attempting to understand "life." But our *understanding* of life processes (i.e., our representations of them) are *not* the processes themselves. Partly because of the structure of our language, we tend to identify one with the other. We treat the map as though it were the territory. And we forget that the map can never cover all the territory, and that it must inevitably reflect the bias, or framework, of whomever made it. And we forget (or learn in spite of ourselves to ignore) a simple truth that infants and animals know: *the territory is more important than the map.* Nature *as given* is more significant for our well-being than our representations of it.

Unfortunately, because the territory for humans is so deeply enmeshed with their maps, it is not always clear how much of what we see is actually there, and how much is a projection of ourselves. For example: John has a headache, he takes a pill that he expects will make it go away, and it does. He says, "The pill cured my headache." But since he *expected* it to cure his headache — was it the pill, or John's expectation that did it? It is difficult for human beings to get away from this "placebo factor" — their representations (their beliefs or "knowledge") of what a remedy, diet, or prescription is *supposed* to do for them, which they learned from reading books or listening to mother or the doctor.

No such problem exists with non-human animals. If a cat is sick and is given a pill and recovers, we can be reasonably confident that the white coat and diploma of the person administering it had little to do with the cure. As for the pill, it may or may not have helped.

It is important to note that many of the same drugs are used for both cats and humans. This is because, genetically, they are cousins, and so often respond similarly to similar types of medicinal or nutritional input. Consequently, there is much of significance for humans in the results of a unique nutritional experiment that was carried out to compare the effects of raw vs. cooked food on cats (and incidentally, on plants). The results carry heavy implications for human well-being, but have largely been ignored by the medical profession (for whom nutrition has generally seemed irrelevant). They corroborate the Anopsological theses that no animal can, without ill effect, ingest food its genetic code is not prepared to metabolize.

The study, carried out over a ten-year period in the 1930s and 1940s, compared the health, skeletal and dental development for two populations of cats. One was fed essentially raw meat scraps, the other cooked meat, with raw milk for both groups (later experiments reversed this to raw milk for one group and cooked milk for others, with raw meat for both):[1]

Cats on Raw Meat Diet

Over their life spans they prove resistant to infections, to fleas and to various other parasites, and show no signs of allergies. In general they are gregarious, friendly and predictable in their behavior patterns and when dropped as much as six feet to test their coordination they always land on their feet and come back for more "play". These cats produce one homogeneous generation after another with the average weight of the kitten at birth being 119 grams. Miscarriages are rare and the litters average five kittens with the mother cat nursing her young without difficulty.

Cats on Cooked Meat Diet

Heart problems; nearsightedness and farsightedness; underactivity of the thyroid or inflammation of the thyroid gland; infections of the kidney, of the liver, of the testes, of the ovaries and of the bladder; arthritis and inflammation of the joints; inflammation of the nervous system with paralysis and meningitis — all occur commonly in these cooked meat fed cats.

Cooked meat fed cats show much more irritability. Some females are even dangerous to handle . . . the males on the other hand are more docile, even to the point of being unaggressive and their sex interest is slack or perverted . . . Vermine and intestinal parasites abound. Skin lesions and allergies appear frequently and are progressively worse from one generation to the next . . . Abortion in pregnant females is common running about 25 percent in the first [cooked meat] generation to about 70 percent in the second. Deliveries are generally difficult with many females dying in labor . . . The average weight of the kittens is 100 grams, 19 grams less than the raw meat nurtured kittens.

Further experiments were made feeding cat groups respectively: raw milk, pasteurized milk and evaporated milk, but with raw meat for all groups. The results corresponded to those for the raw vs. cooked meat experiments. The raw milk cats were generally healthy and resistant to infections and parasites. The pasteurized milk cats showed progressive constitutional and respiratory problems similar to those shown by the cooked meat cats. Cats fed condensed milk showed even more damage than their pasteurized milk counterparts, with the most marked deficiencies occurring in those fed sweetened condensed milk. In an experiment with Vitamin D milk (from cattle fed irradiated yeast), the females seemed unaffected, but the young males did not live beyond the second month, and the adult males died within ten months.

Cows' milk in any form is not an original food for cats, only for calves. Pottenger's cats apparently did well on cows' milk as long as it was raw, but he did not explore the effects of a totally milk-free diet on his animals except by accident, without remarking upon the total absence of milk:

Kittens in which deficiency is established by an inadequate diet show stigmata throughout their lives. If deficient kittens are allowed to live in the open and feed upon rats, mice, birds, gophers and other food natural to the cat, they will show a certain degree of correction in their deficiencies.

In another experiment showing the effects of instinctive feeding (but unrelated to milk), a group of guinea pigs were initially fed a diet of rolled and cracked grain with supplements of cod liver oil and field-dried alfalfa. In a short time they showed loss of hair, paralysis and high litter mortality, with an increase in pneumonia, diarrhea and other deficiency symptoms. When fresh-cut green grass was introduced into their diet, they showed remarkable improvement. A few guinea pigs with severe diarrhea were allowed to run outside the pens to feed on growing grass and weeds. In less than 30 days these animals showed even greater improvement than those receiving fresh-cut greens inside the pens. Their diarrhea stopped, their hair returned with a soft, shiny, velvety texture, and they healed and became well, with no recurrence of gastrointestinal upset or other ailments.

In fact a partial correction of many deficiencies and a healing of disease symptoms is exactly what happens to humans when they eat only native food – when they "forage" by instinct among a variety of raw original foods. We should not really be surprised.

The Pottenger experiments included a comparison of the effects on cats of consuming milk from range-fed cows or cows fed dry grasses and industrial by-products such as molasses, cotton seed meal, or grape pulp. He found that cats fed raw milk from feed-lot cows showed the same defects as those fed pasteurized milk. He went on to compare farm chickens that were free to eat worms, grasses and weeds, with hatchery chickens housed in wire pens and fed dry feeds. The former laid eggs with hard shells and deep yellow yolks, from which husky, healthy chicks hatched. In contrast, hatchery chickens laid thin-shelled eggs with pale yolks, a large percentage of which failed to germinate when fertilized. The farm chickens contained twice as much calcium as the mass-produced ones.

Obviously, a price will be paid by any creature, human or otherwise, that eats food not intended for it, or that was not itself nourished on original food for *it*. The representations produced by laboratory analyses, of the "content" of a food, are misleading for determining the needs of living organisms in the real world.

> *In comparing the diets of farm and hatchery chickens and of range and dry feed lot cattle, we find that they all contain adequate amounts of fat, protein, carbohydrates and minerals.* The difference lies in the presence or absence of fresh factors. *It is the fresh, raw factors in feed that appear to hold the balance between a healthy animal capable of reproducing healthy offspring and one that is unhealthy and has poor reproductive efficiency. Logically, the nutritional value of animal products such as milk and eggs depends on the nutritional value of the producing animals' diet.*

Pottenger did several experiments raising navy beans in separate plots of ground fertilized with the excreta of cats fed raw or cooked food. The plants were compared for germination rates, growth rates, size and appearance. The raw-food excreta fertilized plants did well, while plants grown with cooked-food fertilizer did poorly (plants in an unfertilized plot gave intermediate results). The greatest contrast appeared in the beans themselves:

> *RAW MEAT: These beans have a hard, white surface. Uniformity of size and plumpness of the beans distinguishes them from the beans of all other groups.*

> *COOKED MEAT: In this group, one-fourth of the beans are shriveled and yellow in color; the remainder are smooth and white. They also are more plump than the milk beans, but they are not as plump as the raw meat beans. They exhibit the peculiar oblong shape of the milk beans.*

It should be evident that when animals, man included, or plants, ingest foods to which they are not adapted, abnormalities will occur. It should also be evident that the genetic code of each living organism is prepared to properly metabolize and make use only of the foods it is "familiar with" from the millions of years of its evolutionary past. But we are not familiar with "Vitamin C" and "Vitamin B₁₂" and "Zinc" and "Iron" and "Amino Acids". Our bodies do indeed require some variable amounts of the molecules these verbal abstractions refer to. But we do not require them as isolated entities packaged in separate bottles because it is convenient to market them that way. They are never separate in nature. The whole is more than the sum of its parts. A peach is more than "fructose" + "fiber" + "Vitamin C" + "water", and we did not become genetically adapted to its analyzable parts, we evolved in relationship to the unified *whole*, "fresh factor" included.

> *An analysis of a dead body and an analysis of a handful of soil will show them to both be composed of the same elements, but no one can mistake the flesh of a man for a handful of soil. An apple too is made up of the same elements as the soil, but we easily recognize the vast difference between this product of vital synthesis and the soil in our garden.* [2]

All of which is to say, in summary, that plants and animals (ourselves included) were built to thrive on the foods nature prepared for them, but not necessarily on what *we* might prepare for them.

---

[1] Francis M. Pottenger, Jr., *Pottenger's Cats*, The Price-Pottenger Nutrition Foundation, San Diego, 1983.
[2] Herbert M. Shelton, *The Science and Fine Art of Food and Nutrition*, Natural Hygiene Press, Oldsmar, 1984.

Chapter 6

A Question of Adaptation

It is sometimes argued that men must have become adapted to denatured foods because if they weren't, as a species, they wouldn't have survived to this day. True? Not true? The question warrants exploring.

The genetic mutation of any species both produces and results from changes in the overall structure of the biological plenum. Various models exist to explain how mutations may occur and become self-perpetuating. All point to the conclusion that "life" is an on-going experiment, and that any species that does not mutate in such a way as to adapt to its changing environment will perish. Note that *adaptation* is not synonymous with *adjustment*. Adaptation implies organic structural changes, while adjustment refers to a species or individual coping "as-is" with novel circumstances.

There is no doubt that we can *adjust* to non-original foods – at a price. Are we *adapted* to them however? In order to explore this, let us first take a brief look at the mechanisms of evolutionary change.

There are many opinions as to how, where and when Homo Sapiens got its start. One of them, advanced by the French paleontologist Yves Coppens' holds that the genealogical branching of man from monkeys possibly began as the result of a cataclysmic geological upheavel around the year 5,000,000 B.C. The abrupt formation of an enormous canyon, the Riff Valley of Ethiopia, would have isolated groups of apes to the east of it from those to the west. Those to the west would have continued to live happily in the tropical rain forest environment to which they had become adapted over the preceding twenty million years. The ones to the east, however, would have found themselves in an environment that was beginning to dry out. As rainfall diminished, so would the density of plant life, and the ability to climb trees for food would become less important for survival than the ability to cover long distances. Speed, keen eyesight, and cunning, would also have become more critical for survival than they were in the jungle. Consequently, the individuals with the strongest legs, the best eyes and the biggest brains would have been the ones best able to survive and reproduce, passing these characteristics on to succeeding generations.

This example might lead us to assume that evolutionary adaptation is quite a simple and straightforward process, unless we realize the time-spans involved. For the evolutionary road leading to Homo Sapiens is so long that it is practically beyond our understanding. Humankind's oldest recorded history goes back only a few thousand years, and the archeological remains of "ancient" civilizations are hardly any older. For most of us, however, the "dawn of civilization" happened too long ago to even try to think back to. The 200 odd years that have elapsed since the creation of the United States already seems like a "very long time" to most of us. So we have trouble grasping the fact that men and women very much like ourselves were already walking the earth not only 2,000 or 20,000 years ago, but 200,000 and 2,000,000,000 years and more into the past. Already, five *million* years ago, our ancestors had come down from the trees and one generation after another, were changing in response to their changing environment, becoming finally ourselves, in the world we live in today.

Ten thousand years at most have elapsed since our ancestors first began to plant seeds and keep domestic animals. Over millions of years before inventing agriculture they were hunters and gatherers – they ate whatever they could find, and wandered elsewhere when food was scarce. Paleontological remains indicate that in some areas they began to cook meat as early as 400,000 B.C.; in others, it was not until a quarter of a million years later. But in terms of evolutionary time-spans, 250,000 years ago is "yesterday," and 10,000 years is "a moment ago." So we have to ask: assuming the human race could in theory become adapted to the molecular alimentary innovations wrought by cooking and husbandry – *has it had time* to do so?

Homo Sapiens' parental apes could not have been adapted to milk, bread or roast beef simply because, over the 70,000,000 years of *their* evolutionary development, such foods as these were *never* part of their diet. Monkeys today can presumably *adjust* to such foods in captivity (with consequences similar to those for men), but *adapted* they are certainly not. What about us?

Men and monkeys are very, *very* similar in many important respects. The structure of the digestive tracts of men and chimpanzees (our nearest genetic cousins) is practically the same. We carry the same sorts of intestinal flora, and many of the same viruses. We harbor many of the same parasites and diseases. And it turns out that our genetic codes are almost identical.

Various approaches have been used for determining the "genetic distance" between species. Comparisons have been made between men and monkeys using behavioral, anatomical, physiological and other criteria. On molecular levels, the determination involves a structural comparison of their DNA. DNA is our cellular "information system," containing the instructions for our

reproductive and metabolic processes, and for practically everything else that goes on in our bodies. The amount of information it contains is enormous. Figuratively speaking, the DNA in
a single cell holds as much "data," coded electro-chemically, as
the books in a public library. It is encoded in the form of a dou-
ble helix whose sequential molecular arrangement is peculiar to
each species. The amount of DNA in our bodies is far from
negligible, for if a length of DNA from one cell were to be un-
coiled and stretched out straight, it would be nearly three feet
long. With our billions of cells, we each contain, so to speak,
enough DNA to stretch around the world fifty or sixty times.

> . . . some of the amino acid sequences in humans were virtually
> identical with those of apes such as the chimpanzee or gorilla.[2]

> . . . the sequences of human and chimpanzee polypeptides examined
> to date are, on the average, more than 99 percent identical.[3]

The DNA from a chimp, compared point to point with the
DNA from a human, differs by 1.1% overall. This is to say that
two three-foot lengths of human and chimpanzee DNA laid side
by side fail to match one another over only one four-tenths of
an inch of their length.

It may not be correct to assume that the differentiation between man and chimpanzees has been growing at a steady rate,
because some "quantum jump" mutations may well have occurred
along the way. But if we assume a steady evolutionary rate, then
the gulf between men and chimpanzees has been widening at
the rate of only twenty-two one-hundredths of one percent *per
million years*. So that in the 400,000 years (at most) since man began using fire for cooking, *less than 1/10th of one percent* of his DNA
code could potentially have evolved in response to the novel nutritional molecules so produced.

The human genetic constitution has changed relatively little since the appearance of truly modern human beings, Homo sapiens sapiens, about 40,000 years ago. Even the development of agriculture 10,000 years ago has apparently had a minimal influence on our genes.[4]

Furthermore, for a mutation to occur or a characteristic to become emphasized in response to some changed factor in the environment, that factor would have to be constant — which would not be the case with cooked foods, since different foods cooked in different manners at different temperatures for different lengths of time would necessarily produce different thermally generated compounds. So that positive adaptation to specific heat-modified foods could hardly have taken place.

Such developments as the Industrial Revolution, agribusiness, and modern food-processing techniques have occurred too recently to have had any evolutionary effect at all. Accordingly, the range of diets available to preagricultural human beings determines the range that still exists for men and women living in the 20th century — the nutrition for which human beings are in essence genetically programmed.[5]

[1] Yves Coppens, *Le Singe, l'Afrique et l'Homme,* Fayard, Paris 1983.
[2] Mary-Claire King and A. C. Wilson, "Evolution at Two Levels in Humans and Chimpanzees", *Science,* Vol. 188 No. 4184, April 11, 1975.
[3] Ibid.
[4] From *Paleolithic Nutrition* by S.B. Eaton and M. Konner, The New England Journal of Medicine, Jan., 1985.
[5] Ibid.

Chapter 7

How to "Civilize" Food

Part I: Cooking and Chemistry

How can you explain our drive, unique among living things, to convert whatever natural thing we touch, into something that never existed before . . .?

For transforming food we learned to use fire, coals and hot stones, skewers, leave wrappings, pots and pans and covers for them . . . pressure cookers, gas and electric and micro-wave ovens, infra-red radiators . . .

For cooking is the most effective and radical way by far to modify food. Heat speeds up the movements of food's atoms, disturbs their electrostatic bonds, accelerates their interactions. It creates new chemical compounds; it creates molecules that did not exist before.

However, cooking is not generally thought of as chemistry. It is not called a science, it is known as an art. In the kitchen it is legitimate to add a "spoonful" of X, a "pinch" of Y, a "handful" of Z and a "cup" of Q to roughly two pounds of K, and raise the temperature to "medium" for an hour or so. Any laboratory chemist who operated in these terms would be fired on the spot.

Cooking can be regulated, as it is in assembly-line kitchens, so that each batch of cooked product contains carefully measured amounts of the same types of ingredients. This may ensure uniform quality, but the manufacturer will be eager to point out that the aroma arising from each and every one of his million cans a day is due to somebody's art.

The major difference between a kitchen and a laboratory is that in the latter we know what's going on. Whatever the outcome, we know it came from specific compounds mixed under specific conditions at known temperatures. In a kitchen, however, we simply have no means of analyzing the chemical compounds produced by the interactions between the proteins, acids, fats, starches, salts and oils, in some beef (whose tissues probably also contain hormones, vaccines, fertilizer and pesticide residues), and onions, tomatoes, garlic, salt, pepper, Bay leaf and corn oil — all brought together for an hour or two at a simmer.

We may feel, with some justification, that the type of analysis that concerns us in the kitchen is of another kind. If it smells good — if it tastes good — that's what counts. We may take care to "undercook" our vegetables so as not to destroy the vitamins (and then take a few synthetic ones just in case) but generally our precautions end there. Since we have eaten cooked foods all our lives, they seem as "natural" as the air we breathe. We are not concerned about possible chemical changes because we can hardly conceive that they even took place at all.

Yet no laboratory is needed to tell us they did.

The sensations of smell and taste are produced by molecules from outside the body coming into contact with receptor cells in the nose and tongue. Within our nasal passages, the olfactory epithelium contains some 10 million cells that are constantly in touch with the air we breathe. An even greater number are found in the tongue, and respond to molecules reaching them in an acqueous medium in our mouths.

Any particular smell or taste we experience depends on the structure of the incoming molecules (It also depends on the molecular state of the organism, an issue discussed elsewhere). Even a slight change in structure, which does not affect the molecule's composition (i.e., its chemical formula), may dramatically alter its interactions with its surroundings. Both molecules pictured below have the same number of radicals, but they are placed differently. The trans-p-Menth-8-ene on the left smells like oranges. The cis-p-Menth-8-ene on the right smells like crude oil. Unless analyzed by stereo-chemical methods — OR our noses! — they are chemically "the same."

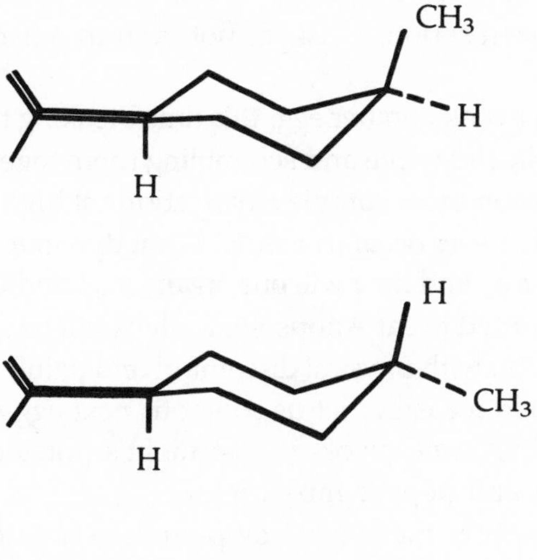

Figure 1
(Stereochemical comparison)

The *new smell* from a stew made from the ingredients mentioned above is due to molecules having a *new structure* reaching receptor cells in our noses. No single ingredient smelled that way at the outset, nor did the original uncooked collection of them. The stew's new taste is unlike the taste of any single ingredient within it, and is also due to molecules having a new structure coming into contact with receptor cells on our tongues.

The novel smell and taste of any cooked food is the product of *molecular structures not found in nature.* For the most part we find them attractive — otherwise, what would have been the point in concocting them in the first place? But we are not genetically prepared for them. While our organisms can manufacture only a limited number of enzymes to break down ingested molecular structures to render them useable, our culinary ingenuity is capable of creating unlimited numbers of new ones that are unknown to our biochemical makeup.

Let us fry an egg on a dry skillet and watch the albumin turn white, and we wonder — what is happening to its structure? No one really knows. Every time we ever watched an egg turn white we were dealing with "cooking," not "chemistry," so the question has never been seriously asked, not even in our research institutions.

Now let's cook another egg, this time breaking the membrane between yolk and white and scrambling them together. Here we are getting even more complex interactions at high temperature, which would never occur in nature. What dynamic structures are they producing, and how will our organisms handle them? (Once you have learned to eat Anopsologically you'll be able to answer that one easily: with physical discomfort and pain!) And just once more for good measure: let us cook our next egg with some oil on the skillet, some pieces of last night's potatoes, and some cheese, salt and pepper mixed in.

This time how many new compounds of unknown structure did we create? We really don't know, but assuming we browned the potatoes:

> . . . *the number of derivatives appearing at the end is extremely impressive; we are constantly discovering new ones: volatile alco-*

> hols, cetones, aldehydes, esters, ethers, non-volatile heterocycles.
> The overall result is a mixture of derivatives with different chemi-
> cal and biological properties: aromatic, peroxydizing, anti-oxydizing,
> toxic, some of them possibly mutagenic or carcinogenic and even
> anti-mutagenic and anti-carcinogenic. As an indication, at the pres-
> ent time in a fried potato we have identified more than 50 deriva-
> tives, most of them derivatives of pyrozenes and thiazole; but we
> know that in all, there are still 400 yet to be identified.[1]

It is not our aim to alarm anyone, except regarding the state
of our ignorance. Our best known writers in medicine, nutrition,
and dietetics, usually fail to distinguish between raw and cooked
food except in limited terms of nutrients lost or destroyed. And
when "nutritional value" is discussed, it is not always clear what
values are being referred to.

Let us put it this way: when a child gets lost, he knows where
he is, it's his parents who don't. When we "lose" nutrients in
the pot, it's not that they've vanished into thin air (although some
volatile ones may effectively be carried away), but rather that
they've combined with others to make new kinds of molecules.
They've gone where we can't find them any longer. A food's
"nutritional value" may in effect be destroyed or "lost," but it is
its *value* that is so affected, not the molecules themselves. They
do not cease to exist, but become transformed in ways that neither our laboratories nor our enzymes can identify.

> In general terms the premelanoidins formed during the first stages
> (of roasting meat) are not digestible and even have negative effects
> on the digestibility of the unaltered proteins and on protein effi-
> ciency.[2]

All of this is to say that cooking and chemistry might usefully be thought of together. Raising the temperature of a food
changes its molecular structure. At the least, we will eat it to excess
because denatured food will not trigger an alliesthetic (taste-
change) reaction to protect us from eating more than we need,
leading to a toxic overload. But we will also be ingesting toxic
compounds the food did not contain in its original state.

Just for emphasis, let us briefly take a look at the kind of "cooking" (i.e., chemistry) done not in skillets, but in commercial kitchen-factories whose products fill so much of our supermarket shelf-space. We will consider just one product, a popular type of cookie. The recipe is somewhat different from the one familiar to girl scouts; it contains at the outset *no natural ingredients at all* — except possibly whole eggs (if they were actually added straight from the shell, which is doubtful). According to the label, the cookies contained before being processed:

Cottonseed oil, soybean oil, beef or pork fat, unbleached flour, Vitamin A, Vitamin D, ferrous sulphate, thiamine, niacin, riboflavin, sugar, skim milk, cocoa, dextrose, egg yolks, soya flour, starch, sodium acid pyrophosphate, baking soda, sodium aluminum phosphate, fumaric acid, salt, toasted ground wheat, rye flour, corn flour, potato flour, whole eggs, egg whites, guar gum, karaya gum, dextrin, lecithin, polysorbate 60, sodium stearol-2-lactylate, sodium caseinate, mono- and dyglycerides, propylene glycol mono and diesters, whey, spice, artificial colors, artificial flavor, and corn syrup.

Merely baking this mixture would produce recompounded chemical structures of indescribable complexity, alien to our metabolisms. But in the factory, even further denaturation is in order first. In order to increase its market appeal, the mixture will be "texturized" by a process that deliberately causes the macromolecules in the ingredients to lose their native organization and structure. The batter will be sent to a "pre-conditioner" to be "pre-cooked," then extruded through a device where it will again be heated by mechanical torsion and possibly even injected steam:

> . . . *which transforms it into a viscous, plasticized material whose denatured molecules can recombine at their exposed electrostatic, hydrogen, covalent and ionic bonding sites.*[3]

We are incapable even of imagining, let alone determining by analysis, all the kinds of molecular novelties such methods produce. We should only marvel that the product is labelled "food."

But we need not go to even a fraction of this trouble to denature food. Even slight increases in temperature may modify a food's molecular structure enough to make it impossible to evaluate instinctively. For example, it is common commercial practice to heat honey in order to remove it from the honeycomb and/or make it easier to pour into jars. Our taste-change mechanism will not function correctly with honey so treated. Original honey sooner or later "burns" the palate to stop us from eating any more. Denatured honey does not. It can be eaten to excess, producing nausea, "allergic" reactions, and a wealth of other symptoms.

Other seemingly "natural" foods may also be denatured by inadvertent cooking. There is practically no dried fruit of any sort on the commercial market today that has not at some stage of production been heated well above its native ambient temperature. In some cases it is done to save time, in others to prevent fungus or bacteria from growing. By treating the fruit with boiling water, drying it in ovens or irradiating it, the producers unwittingly increase demand for their product, because even if the fruit is not rendered patently toxic (which is unfortunately often the case), it will fail to trigger a taste change, allowing far more to be eaten than was needed. Dates, bananas or any other fruit may indeed be "good for us," but only in the proper amounts. Too much of a "good" thing is no longer good at all.

However we go about it, heat produces chemical changes in food. It kills cells — bacteria among others — of which we have been taught to be afraid (so we end up eating dead bacteria). But it also kills cells in the food itself, so we end up eating dead food. By adding seasoning and other ingredients, we are in effect attempting to give it "life" as we kill it. But the result is further chemical change for which our biochemical makeup is not prepared. Instinctively we know this: cooked food that is merely cooked, that is unmixed or unseasoned, holds no interest for our palates.

> *Looking for an explanation for this more dramatic improvement in the guinea pigs feeding on the fresh growing grasses and weeds, we noticed that when we put our arms inside the sacks of cut grass, the temperature inside was warmer than the temperature outside. It proved to range between five degrees and 30 degrees warmer. This suggests that the cut grass becomes semi-cooked by the time it reaches the guinea pigs, and that important, thermolabile substances are at least partly destroyed.[4]*

> *High temperature cooking and sterilization . . . may change the ionic value of metals, so that minerals may be present in food after cooking but are not useable by the body.[5]*

[1] *Pyrolyse des Aliments et Risques de Toxicite*, R. Derache, Cahiers de Nutrition et de Dietetique, Vol. XVII, 1982.

[2] *Consequences Nutritionnelles de la Cuisson par les Micro-Ondes*, Araudo & Sorbier, Ibid.

[3] *Extrusion Texturization of Foods* by J. W. Harper, Food Technology, Vol 40, No. 3, 1986.

[4] Francis M. Pottenger, *Pottenger's Cats*, The Price-Pottenger Nutrition Foundation, San Diego, 1983.

[5] Schutte & Meyers, *Metabolic Aspects of Health*, Discovery Press, Kentfield, CA, 1979.

Chapter 8

How to "Civilize" Food

Part II: Non-cooking and Chemistry

Does our drive to modify foods reflect only a desire to enoble them, that they might in turn enoble whomever shall eat them? . . . But food in its native state is as noble as it will ever be, and by our hand we can only degrade it. Aside from baking and roasting, boiling and toasting, let us briefly consider a few other things we know how to do to food, besides eat it.

Freezing

As it was explained briefly in Chapter 4, "Fresh-frozen" food may indeed have been fresh before freezing, but afterwards it is not.

63

When water freezes with organic tissues, it expands, rupturing cell membranes to produce submicroscopic mixtures unknown in nature. The diminished smell and taste of frozen food is evidence of the food's denatured structure.

Frozen food will not produce an alliesthetic (taste-change) response to protect the organism from consuming more than it needs. Furthermore, most frozen foods are washed, or treated with boiling water, before being frozen. This also contributes to its denaturation.

Simply cooling fish or meat with ice (which does not freeze it) does not denature it to any significant degree. However, even ice will quickly damage many kinds of vegetable produce — which gives some indication of how deep-freezing affects them.

Extracts

The juice from a fruit or vegetable does not include everything the food contained in its original form, and particularly, the whatever-it-is in original food that produces an alliesthetic response to protect against overloads. Organic fluids, such as oils from grains, seeds, and olives, may contain useful nutrients as defined by laboratory analysis, but they are not whole foods. Because they can easily be consumed to excess, they may become toxic.

In some cases, extraction processes involve heating (see above). The most widely consumed extract is *sugar*: whether "raw" or "refined," it bears little kinship to the original cane or beets whose juices were used to produce it. Packaged fructose, a dehydrated extract from fruit that may structurally be more akin to the original, is not a "natural" sugar either in the Anopsological sense.

Extracts from whole foods also are exposed to the air and may also become toxic as a consequence.

Dehydrating

Most commercially dehydrated products are subjected to high temperature at some stage of production, and will not trigger a taste change when eaten. Fresh peppers, for example, will be good for the organism if they taste good, but their effect cannot be predicted once they are dried and powdered. (In excess, they will be toxic.) Once dehydrated food powders have been exposed to the air, they become further altered by oxydation.

Concentrates may be convenient to use, but they are not natural foods. Diluted orange juice concentrate is not an orange. "Instant" mashed potatoes are not potatoes. Soaked onion flakes cannot again a whole onion make.

Foods that are dried at their native ambient temperature retain the ability to trigger an alliesthetic response, but are rarely available in commerce. A discussion of home drying can be found in Chapters 21 and 22.

Mixing

This is where the advocates of raw and "living" foods (among others) usually miss the point. It is generally believed that salads provide healthy and desirable nourishment. Salads may also provide much undesirable nourishment because we are unable to evaluate the taste of more than one food in our mouth at a time. When our body needs raw onions, they will taste sweet, like cherries, reverting to a biting taste when we have had our fill. When mixed with tomatoes, cucumbers, salt, oil, and vinegar, we will not know when to stop (or recognize our need for some other vegetable in the concoction that we do in fact need). Mixing sugar and/or cream with strawberries will enable us to ingest more strawberries than our body needs, which may produce an "allergic" reaction.

Note that commercially bottled honey is more often than not a mixture of honeys from different sources (that were probably heated to facilitate handling). Such honey will not produce an alliesthetic response.

Grinding

Chopping or grinding a food destroys its structural integrity and does so in an oxygen environment rather than the saliva-filled environment of our mouths. Processed raw foods such as grated carrots or uncooked hamburger ("Tartar steak") if eaten at once will generally produce a mild alliesthetic response, but can easily be eaten to excess unless close attention is paid to the taste.

Pickling and Salting

Pickling is an effective means of preserving foods at room temperature, and imparting a taste that some people enjoy. Once a person has adjusted to instinctive eating, he will probably find the taste of pickled or salted foods too strong to be attractive. A similar remark applies to smoked foods, which he is likely to find taste . . . like smoke!

Washing and Polishing

When fruits or vegetables are washed, polished, waxed, and so forth as they often are in modern supermarkets, it becomes impossible to tell by smell whether or not we need (i.e., want) them. The widespread use of pesticides makes it generally mandatory to do some cleaning, or remove the skin entirely before eating. But we may be paying a price for our obsession with "cleanliness:"

> *It is almost certain that a good supply of mineral elements was supplied to the people who ate raw foods directly from the ground without washing them. A coating of earth-dust on carrots, turnips,*

potatoes, tomatoes and other vegetables when eaten raw, was a good
source of mineral nutrition.'

When seafoods or meat are washed, most of the smell and taste are lost, inevitably along with a good part of the nutritional value. A fish may be rinsed before being cut open, but afterwards should be wiped clean only, without water.

It will be argued that washing food is necessary to safeguard against dirt, worms, amoebas, or other "infectious agents" it might be carrying. This is undoubtedly true to a great extent for "normally" nourished people with high toxicity levels and dormant immunological responses, but once a person has begun eating instinctively on a regular basis, he need not worry too much about them. But note: *on a regular basis.*

Non-human Food

Any food that could not be consumed by human beings a million years ago (before we mastered fire, discovered cooking or invented ropes and pots) cannot truly be food for us now. There are two major types of non-foods for humans that we mistakenly consume with detrimental effects: *dairy products and cooked cereals.* Both are discussed more thoroughly in Chapters 17 and 28. Corn (maize) is an exception, since it can be eaten with pleasure in its original state, fresh from the stalk.

Pollutants

Chemical fertilizers, herbicides, and pesticides, necessarily find their way into the plants they are used on, and eventually into us. The same applies to hormones, vaccines, antibiotics and other substances given to animals. Coloring agents, sweeteners, and preservatives added to food during processing, also share in producing an unhealthy population.

The use of "organic" compost does not fully answer the problem of chemical fertilizers, and deserves special comment. Compost heaps, decomposed by anaerobic bacteria, may rise to very high temperatures, and like ovens, produce novel chemical compounds – particularly when the heap contains cooked-food remains to begin with. (Please see the reference to Pottenger's bean experiments in Chapter 5.)

Artificial Breeding and Hybridization

Most current varieties of fruits and vegetables were bred by artificial selection to develop particular qualities of color, resistance to fungus or parasites, freezability, taste, shelf-life, size, rate of growth, mildew resistance, texture, appearance, etc. (but rarely for their nutritional qualities). Strictly speaking, they are not true original foods: commercially bred fruits and vegetables do not produce the strong, clear-cut alliesthetic reactions wild ones do. Generally speaking, fruits are bred to taste good when raw, vegetables to taste good when cooked. What this means for people who eat them raw is that they will generally find fruit *over*-attractive, vegetables *under*-attractive. They may want to compensate accordingly, eating vegetables until their taste becomes strongly unattractive, but stopping with fruit when it becomes only mildly unpleasant. This point is discussed in Chapter 23.

Irradiation

Irradiating food kills parasites, and fungi but is employed primarily because it increases its shelf life. It is particularly significant that irradiation *prevents produce from ripening,* in other words, it kills it. When and if irradiation of fresh food becomes widespread, the majority of U.S. city dwellers will no longer have original, genetically adapted foods available to them at all. Some new and fascinating forms of pathology will doubtless appear as a result.

Remember that cows fed irradiated yeast (although the "irradiation" is of another kind) produce "Vitamin D Milk" that makes cats sick, and produces abnormal beans on plants fertilized with their excrement (please see Chapter 5).

An added danger arises from the fact that produce may legally be irradiated without any notice given to the consumer. Irradiation affects foods just as strongly as any chemical preservative.

Other considerations

There is little doubt that some things have been omitted here, or that something new will come along that will do strange and wonderful things to food that nature never thought of.

"Naturally" denatured foods, almost but not quite "the real thing," eaten individually and infrequently, may do relatively little harm. But when a diet includes practically nothing else, it can be extremely dangerous to one's health. When nature is paid an insult, she tends to pay it back.

Fortunately, as we will see in the following chapters, the same holds true for compliments.

' Schutte & Meyers, *Metabolic Aspects of Health,* Discovery Press, Kentfield CA, 1979.

PART II
FOOD, HEALTH AND ILLNESS

Chapter 9

How Food Produces Illness

Digestively speaking, humans, hogs and rats are the planet's most versatile species. They are the ambulatory garbage dumps of the animal kingdom, and can eat practically any denatured food and survive long enough to reproduce. As zoo keepers can testify, almost any wild animal fed denatured foods will quickly become sick and die, poisoned by unnatural molecules it is unable to process. But humans, along with the pigs and rats that eat their leftovers, are generally able to adjust – for a time.

For a time only, however, and not in all cases, and at a price. So much of their energy must be devoted to cleaning up the molecular garbage they ingest, that relatively little is left over for other tasks.

This problem has generally gone unnoticed. In order to explore it, we have deliberately coined the term "Intoxination"

73

(with "n") to designate poisons not usually thought of as poisons, which strain the organism's ability to flush itself clean. We will come back to this point in a moment.

The current medical notion of *Intoxication* (with "c") refers to poisoning the body with chemicals, drugs, and gasses (artificially produced for the most part), or bacteria, venom, recognized toxic foods (e.g., toadstools, spoiled meat or accumulated metabolic wastes). "Detoxication" (or "detoxification") refers to eliminating these types of poisons or rendering them harmless.

But the usual notion of toxic substances fails to take account of the alien (and demonstrably toxic) molecules contained in denatured food. So we are using the term "IntoxiNation" to denote the unrecognized poisoning produced by the altered molecular structure of non-original foods (whose denaturation is generally perceived in our culture as "normal" or even "natural" for humans). We will occasionally refer to the poisons themselves as "NUtoxins" (for nutritional).

A corollary, "DetoxiNation," will be used in reference to the elimination of nutoxins from the body. Detoxination often occurs in ways, and via channels, that are not recognized for what they are (a cleansing, health-restoring process). Consequently, the symptoms of detoxination are more often than not classified as an "illness," and efforts are made to suppress them, frequently with drugs. Tragically, as drugs halt the cleaning-out process, they intoxicate the body even further. This may in turn cause other new symptoms to appear (that again constitute detoxination or detoxification phenomena, again not recognized as such) leading again to new attempts to suppression with drugs, in a vicious cycle, producing "iatrogenic" (caused by drugs) disease.

Detoxinaton is a natural and necessary process that occurs spontaneously if not interfered with. Even though our remote, prehistoric ancestors might have been eating only native foods to which they were genetically adapted, they would also have been ingesting any number of things their bodies couldn't use and would need to eliminate, such as: dirt, worms, insects, bacteria, fungi, and other animals' excreta. They would also have been eating food that was not in a pristine original condition, such as a partially decomposed carcass or fish, or a fallen fruit that had baked in the sun. Consequently, their genetic code necessarily included instructions for eliminating the toxins these less-than-perfect foods contained – just as ours does today. Barring accidents, they would have been protected against truly poisonous foods by their senses of smell and taste, since dangerous substances in nature generally carry an unattractive or repellent odor, and their taste is disagreeable.

Should there be any doubt that we are daily ingesting huge amounts of unnatural chemical compounds, let us remember that the novel smells of cooked foods (among others) *mean* novel molecules. The sensation of smell is the result of specific air-borne molecules striking specialized sensor cells in our noses, which then react by sending electrical signals to our brains, where the sensation we call "smell" actually happens. This mechanism is extremely sensitive. In some cases, fewer molecules may suffice to trigger a smell sensation than can even be detected by laboratory instruments.

We do not generally realize how much just a little can do. Very minute amounts of a substance, even in the form of a vapor, may have overwhelming effects on our bodies. A millionth of a gram of chloroform can knock a 150-pound adult unconscious. The ingestion of as little as 1/500,000 gram of a botulism toxin can be fatal. Numerous chemicals in undetectable or barely detectable amounts can cause blindness, paralysis or death (and particularly in the case of man-made molecules, they may carry no smell at all).

Homeopathic remedies demonstrate how dramatic effects on the body may be produced by amounts of chemicals so minute that it is impossible even to detect their presence. In fact, in some cases, the *fewer* there are, the *greater* their effect.

You may find it difficult to realize just how potent "almost nothing" can be. But consider how homeopathic preparations, for example, are typically made by dilutions. One drop of a saturated solution of a chemical agent is mixed with 100 drops of distilled water in a recipient; then a single drop of this new solution is mixed with 100 drops of distilled water in another recipient; then one drop of this newly diluted solution is mixed with 100 times its volume in another recipient, and so on as many as 15 times. If you will divide one by a hundred, by a hundred, and then again ten or fifteen times, you will begin to see what this means. You might even wish to experiment, starting with one drop of india ink in a hundred drops of water, and seeing how far you get before the color disappears.

By the fifteenth dilution — and in fact, well before — the amount of the original substance is "gone," and yet, its effect on the body may often be greater in the higher dilutions than in the lower. So it should not surprise us that very small numbers of unknown molecules from our everyday menu, undetectable by laboratory methods (either because there are so few present, or because we do not know what to look for) can produce significant symptoms.

And surprising as it may seem, even though sophisticated laboratory instruments and procedures may be unable to detect these novel compounds, our noses usually can.

The reason is simple:

When diets are restricted to native foods only, in their original, unmodified state, *human beings and animals carry practically no odors at all.* Their urine, feces, sweat, breath, sputum, vaginal discharges, etc., *do not smell.* It is only when ingested substances are incompletely metabolized that they carry a smell.

What this means in practical terms is that after eating only original foods instinctively for a time, you will not have bad breath, your unwashed feet will not stink, and your excrement will be odorless.

Let us try to better understand what it means if a person *does* carry odors.

Assume you have been practicing instinctive nutrition long enough to become free of smells. Then suddenly smells reappear. The only reasons can be: 1) either you are discharging (detoxinating) unnatural wastes from some non-original food you just ate, or 2) you are flushing out (detoxinating) remnants from non-original food you ate in the past. When this happens, your odors will tell you what it is you just ate — or what it was that had accumulated in your body from whatever you ate years ago, or regularly over many years — that is now finding its way out (which also applies to medicines).

For example, let us say you have been regularly eating by instinct and have become free of odors. Then on an impulse one evening you eat some roasted peanuts (instead of raw ones). A day or two later your excrement will smell of roasted peanuts. It will smell exactly the way the peanuts smelled before you ate them, unchanged. And once the roasted peanuts have been eliminated your stool will become odorless again.

The reason is that the body had no use for the "roasted" molecules (whose existence was evidenced by the smell). So they were given through tickets on the B.M. express. As an example:

Some dog owners, presumably concerned about their pet's nutritional balance, may occasionally add a raw egg to his diet. Their intentions are good: they want Fido healthy and happy. But they will probably fail to notice, when Fido next does his thing, that he leaves upon the sidewalk or in the yard, gooey, transparent egg-white that is in the very same state it was when he ate it. This is because dogs do not possess the enzymatic wherewithall to break down and metabolize egg-white. It passes through their intestinal tract without affecting the dog or vice-versa.

Similarly, human beings do not possess the enzymatic or other wherewithall to metabolize roasted peanuts. We know their original molecular structure was altered because after roasting they carried a new, "roasted" smell. The smell may appeal to us, but it is not a natural attraction. A culinary artifice was used to trick the senses, to make the peanuts smell more attractive than they would have in their original state — and it worked (the technique would not have been adopted if it hadn't). And because they were denatured, we can eat them until we're full, or until we become nauseated or bored with the taste, because no alliesthetic taste-*change* occurs to stop us.

Our metabolisms cannot correctly process roasted peanuts. But some portion of each peanut will have been only *partly* roasted; it will consist of intermediary (semi-cooked) compounds that a human *can* break down and use — *in part*. Some of these compounds, because they are alien only to a degree, may get started through the metabolic process and then get stuck along the way. The system cannot metabolize them completely, so it cannot make full use of them — but neither can it eliminate them as waste (we will see why this is so in a moment). So the incompletely metabolized material will be stored in the cellular vacuoles or elsewhere in the cells, or between them, or in special storage ("fat") cells, until it becomes possible to dislodge them and eliminate them. This event, when it happens, will take the form of a *detoxination sequence* — the second type of circumstance that will cause odors to reappear in a person regularly nourished on native foods.

When a native, natural, genetically appropriate food is eaten, its molecules are first broken down (catabolized) by acids, enzymes, and bacteria, in the stomach and intestinal tract, and are then rebuilt (metabolized) into molecules (metabolites) useable by the cells. The unuseable material in the food, along with cellular wastes, is normally eliminated via the emunctory system, which includes liver, kidneys, intestines, bladder, skin, lungs, tongue, and mucous membranes. The process involves long chain reactions, analogous to a series of chambers behind locked doors, where each molecule is like a key that must be correctly reshaped to fit the next lock if it is to pass through the successive chambers all the way to the end. However, when the food has been denatured (i.e., when its molecular structure is not-quite-right at the outset), it is like a misshapen key, able to go only so far and no further.

Enter the immunological system. The immunological (or "defense") system identifies incoming molecules (either individually or as part of a larger aggregate) as "friends" (to be welcomed) or "foes" (to be rejected), or to put it another way as "like-me" (to be assimilated) or "unlike-me" (to be eliminated). As we will see, in the instinctively fed individual this system will be vigorous and alert, and extremely discerning and intolerant. It will, among other things, insure that not even semi-cooked peanut molecules start through the doors of the metabolism. They will be "sent packing" and be given a chance for so little interaction with the organism that they will emerge smelling exactly the way they smelled when they entered. A vigorous immune system will also destroy and eject any intrusive substance including microbes, amoebas, fungi, tooth fillings, splinters, poisons, etc. along with the body's own mutant cells, as soon as they appear. People with vigorous immune systems (notably, those instinctively nourished) are generally immune to infections, and even to neoplasms.

One of the reasons his immune system will reject not-quite-right peanut material is that the instinctive eater *doesn't need it.* He is well fed, he has all he needs of what *raw* peanuts consist of, he doesn't have to make do with anything less than the real thing. His cells have all the real, nutritive metabolites they need. But beggars can't be choosy. When the nutritionally deficient organism is offered some peanut-material it needs, it will accept it even though it carries with it a load of *mis*-metabolites.

(Imagine that your new pollution-controlled car has run out of gas in some out-of-the-way spot, and all you can find is some old leaded gasoline long stored in a drum. You'll make do with it even though your engine doesn't run smoothly on it, forms sludge and ruins your catalytic converter.)

The pieces of food we put into our mouths, when properly reconstructed by our metabolisms, become molecular "pieces of food" for our cells, called "metabolites." They are our "fuel." But what happens when the fuel is *almost* right but not quite?

In order to visualize how our cells can make only partial use of improperly metabolized molecules, let us simply misconstruct the word "metabolite" itself, and spell it, for instance: EMTABO-LITE (think of the word as representing a molecule, with the individual letters representing the radicals, or atomic clusters, that make it up).

From EMTABOLITE, a denatured sequence of letters, we can extract, by analogy, two linguistically useable bits, "TAB" and "IT," but we have "EM," "SOL" and "E" left over. Alternatively, we could break up the sequence another way, and construct "BITE ME" and "TO," with "A" and "L" left over. But we can't discard the unused letters (just as a molecule can't discard unemployed radicals). And we can't make sense out of *all* the letters except in their natural order. Neither can our bodies process all of a metabolite unless it is "the real thing" and properly constructed, and if it's not, whatever is left over will remain. And over the years, it will accumulate.

With this in mind, we can understand why a "normal" person's immune system will not reject mismetabolites from denatured food as vigorously as someone who eats instinctively.

Early in life, particularly if a baby was breast-fed, his immune system probably did attempt vigorously to eliminate the nutoxins from unnatural foods. Unless mother was a heavy consumer of dairy products before baby was born, when baby was first given cow's milk he probably had some minor diarrhea, vomiting, fever, or rash. The organic complaints were detoxination attempts, but were not understood by the parents or pediatrician, because milk is by definition a "natural and wholesome food" in our society. Of course, no one thought to *smell* the baby. Baby was probably diagnosed as "allergic," and it was expected that the allergy would go away. Probably it did. After being inescapably subjected to cow's milk for a week or two, the immunological system began to tolerate it. (The human organism functions as-a-whole, inseparable from its environment, and its physiological functions are analogous to its psychological ones: it will "put up" with discomforts it can neither flee not fight.)

Shortly, along with the milk, baby began to receive other foods that are supposedly "natural" for babies, such as cooked carrots, spinach, apricots or rhubarb. He probably did not have "allergic" reactions to them, but he *was* occasionally sick with minor symptoms. Had someone with a discerning sense of smell attended to the odors baby exuded at those times, he would have detected: cooked carrots, spinach, apricots, or rhubarb. However, they would not have been clear-cut odors (such as roasted peanuts would produce in an odor-free individual), because within a few months of birth, baby's organism would have become saturated with a variety of mismetabolites that were being eliminated together during the course of his "illness" — along with the ones from the denatured food he was still being fed. So his excrement would smell like . . . excrement.

The mechanism is the same in adults regardless of diet, but when an instinctive eater falls ill, his odors are invariably specific. They can almost always be identified as the odors of denatured foods he ate in the past (but may also include the smells of drugs he was given). So we are led to the inescapable conclusion that an "illness" that produces *unusual smells* must be a *detoxination process* that is eliminating *unusual* (i.e., toxic) *molecules*, regardless of whatever microbial or viral agents are present. Furthermore, under conditions of instinctive nutrition, the symptoms of such illness are much milder than they would be "normally," and their duration much shorter. The reason can only be that the symptoms are actually part of the detoxination process, and when less unnatural food has produced fewer nutoxins, symptoms are correspondingly milder.

Furthermore, in the case of such detoxination "illnesses," if the patient does not go out and immediately reintoxinate himself with denatured food, his health will clearly be better afterwards than it was before. This is strikingly evident for persons who eat regularly by instinct. It means the illness was *useful*. Under conditions of instinctive nutrition it is even common for a person *to be relieved of prior complaints to which the illness was apparently unrelated.*

Under instinctive conditions a Multiple Sclerosis patient will be delighted when he "catches a cold" (a typical detoxination illness), because it promises an improvement in his condition. It is obvious from his odors that his sputum, sweat, urine and feces are carrying with it leftover "T"'s and "A"'s from disordered METABOLITES (see above) that had accumulated in his body. We would not detect them under normal nutritional conditions, because normally the patient would still be ingesting denatured soups, juices, tea, and cooked eggs (to say nothing of drugs used to "treat" the symptoms) whose odors would also be present. Also, the doctor would be unable to detect them because his sense of smell would be desensitized and warped from his own denatured-food eating habits − and perhaps even more importantly: who in their right mind is going to go smelling patients' excreta in the first place?

For someone eating by instinct, any illness whose symptoms are in keeping with the criteria outlined in the next chapter should be looked at as a *health-restoring detoxination process.* It may seem unusual to suggest that some illness, including contagious diseases such as influenza and hepatitis, could be salutary for a person's long-term well-being. But under instinctive nutrition conditions it is clear that they have that effect.

For those suffering from auto-immune or neoplastic pathology, or other "diseases of civilization," it is doubly important that detoxination symptoms be allowed to run their course without being supressed. By enabling the body to redirect energies from garbage detail to construction crew, these symptoms are invaluable aids to self-healing.

The microbes, viruses, or other agents that may be associated with an illness are not its "cause." (The mechanics of viral "infection" are very different from those of microbes, and we will come to them in a moment.) To begin with, the endless numbers of alien microorganisms entering our bodies are, for the most part, destroyed by our immune systems before they can reproduce to any great extent. Only when the immune system is not working properly can their population explode, producing symptoms. But even where particular sets of symptoms are associated with specific types of microorganisms, it does not mean they happened *because* of them. No symptoms would appear if the body didn't *let* them appear; infectious agents alone are not enough.

It is unfortunate that much medical reasoning, even today, is structurally archaic. Medical formulations often still reflect the assumption current in Medieval Europe, that pathology is the work of the Devil. It was believed in the Middle Ages that illness was caused by the Devil, mysteriously entering the body to lodge in the bloodstream. The Devil feared only God, who could hopefully be called to the rescue with prayer. Upon His arrival, the Devil would be frightened away (and the patient would become well again). Today's medical emphasis on "pathogenic agents" − little devils, agents of suffering − that must be destroyed, still reflects this structural assumption. But what about the prior state of the host the agents "invaded?" Such logic takes no account of the *terrain*.

Naive "cause and effect" reasoning has a blinding effect even upon physicians who recognize the multiple factors underlying pathology. Pasteur, who discovered microbes in the first place, advised his peers that they carried less responsibility for disease than the state of the body itself. But his words have too often gone unheeded.

We have explained that *under instinctive nutritional conditions* (but not necessarily under "normal" nutritional conditions), certain illnesses constitute detoxination programs that in fact serve to eliminate denatured-food wastes (as evidenced by their odors). But we can go a step further. We can infer as well that the associated ("pathogenic") microorganisms may in fact be *feeding* upon accumulated mismetabolites that the body would be unable to eliminate without their assistance. For remember that without bacterial help, we would be unable to process even natural food and its wastes in the first place: we carry a greater number of bacteria in our intestinal tracts than cells in our bodies. But our normal flora are not necessarily able to process *unnatural* wastes.

All living organisms are subject to the laws of the survival of the fittest, and infectious microorganisms are no exception. Like other living beings, they mutate and evolve in response to their environments, food sources included. This is how strains of bacteria have emerged that are not only resistant to penicillin or other antibiotics, but that actually thrive on them. So it is not far-fetched at all to infer that some microbes may actually be rendering us a service via their ability to thrive upon mis-metabolized wastes that we would be unable to eliminate without their help.

Consider this:

If a comparison is made between a slice of meat from a steer fed exclusively on grass in a pasture, and free from vaccines and artificially injected hormones, and meat from a steer that ate hay, grains, or industrial fodders it is found that the commercially raised meat begins to turn — begins to harbor a large bacterial population — within two or three days while meat from the animal fed original food will not turn for two to three weeks.

We might even wonder whether a majority of the extraneous microbes found in the world today is better adapted genetically to pollutants than to the absence of pollutants.

This might partially explain why instinctive eaters are immune to infections in cuts and burns (immunological defenses notwithstanding): The infectious "devils" that are adapted to denatured-food toxins can find little or nothing to eat in their absence! And it reflects the fact that an instinctive eater can still become ill with a detoxination "illness" (generally in a benign form) if he has not previously eliminated from his body mismetabolized wastes that the agents of the illness are, in fact, feeding upon (thus breaking them down, which makes their elimination possible).

There are no such things as Lords and Devils, Good Guys and Bad, in the natural world. If humans harbor diseases, there is a reason for them that has nothing to do with evil intent on the part of microscopic "invaders": no creature except man tries to "hurt" another except in order to eat or reproduce. If the microorganisms to which we fall "prey" were not somehow pertinent to our integrity as a species, we would never have evolved so as to attract them to us. Even millions of years ago, there would have been some ingestion of accidentally denatured foods and extraneous material the body could not metabolize or eliminate properly without special help. Fast-mutating germs on the look-out for a meal, and able to quickly adapt to a novel one, would have filled the bill. Kept well in check under instinctive conditions they would not have given rise to acute symptoms.

The same applies to viruses, many of which, even under Anopsological conditions, may also produce detoxination symptoms. Here again the old metaphysics gets in the way when we speak of them as "infectious agents." Viruses are little more than a shell containing DNA or RNA that they inject into a host cell after landing upon its surface. They do not land just anywhere on the cell, however – only at particular sites. And since the cells carry specially prepared landing places for viruses, it is certainly incorrect to speak of a virus "invading" a cell. "Walking in through an open door" is probably more correct.

The DNA or RNA injected by the virus into the cell is nothing more nor less than genetic-code material, i.e., *information*. It is generally said the virus kills the cell "in order to reproduce itself," that it is therefore a "parasite." But that is anthropomorphic language, a projection of our notions of morality and corruption. The virus ceases to exist as an independent entity once it has entered the cell, but stimulates the cell to produce new viruses that emerge and go on to other cells, where the process is repeated.

At some point the process stops (if it didn't, the body's cells would simply be consumed producing new viruses). For a time, however, the viruses spread like messengers bearing instructions, RNA or DNA "program updates" as it were. And it is these instructions that produce the symptoms of influenza, yellow fever, poliomyelitis, or hepatitis. And again, under instinctive nutritional conditions (although not perceptibly under "normal" conditions), these symptoms look like nothing more or less than *detoxination programs*.

Since viruses are produced by cells and reproduced by cells, was it the chicken or the egg that came first? Viruses mutate enormously. In response to what? To mismetabolites in the hosts? They need cellular DNA in order to exist, could the reverse also be true, that our DNA's adjustment or adaptation to a constantly changing environment requires that viral information be available? Might viruses not be thought of as ongoing genetic adaptation experiments on molecular levels? Take, for example, AIDS. It is presumably "incurable." And yet we have seen cases where the symptoms associated with AIDS disappeared once instinctive nutrition had enabled the patient's organism to cleanse itself sufficiently for its immune system to once again gather and properly direct its energies. Would it not therefore be plausible to view the AIDS virus as a very unusual detoxination program for very unusual kinds or amounts of mismetabolites? This may sound too simple to be true, but it might be rewarding to look at it this way.

Of course this is not in line with medical thinking based on Aristotle, Newton and Euclid. But in today's world, a thing can both "be" and "not be," matter is no longer "solid," and lines are no longer "straight." It is time medicine was brought up to date. If it has not yet happened, one of the reasons is – not logic . . . but food. You will understand this once you are eating by instinct. Then, but not before, once your blood and brain have become detoxinated, you will understand that pork-chop- or pancake-based thought is akin to what feeds it. "Mind" is not separate from "body." From the ends of our toes to the tips of our tongues, we are what we eat – ideas and feelings, perceptions and dreams included.

Chapter 10

Symptoms
That Heal

Practically all unpleasant symptoms have been traditionally perceived in medicine as something to be destroyed by executing
the "agent" that "caused" them. One reason for this is that medicine has been ignorant (as we all have) of the toxins in denatured
food. Not realizing they were there, we could not understand
their effects.

But it is now clear that food is a major causative factor in most,
if not all, illnesses. This includes even some conditions not usually
thought of as "abnormal" at all. And it is clear that whatever the
symptoms, their severity directly reflects the degree of intoxination.

In other words, the fewer the nutoxins in the body, the fewer
and/or milder the symptoms, *regardless of any viral, microbial or
other "pathogenic agents" that may be present.* When nutoxins are

at a level that is *truly* "normal" for humans, humans become:

1. *immune to physical pain,*

2. *immune to infections,* and

3. *free of odors* (except when temporarily experiencing a detoxination episode.

These phenomena occur very rarely in people eating the usual "balanced" diets, and almost universally in people eating raw foods selected by instinct.

Although individuals with an extremely *high* level of intoxination may also *seem* free of symptoms as usually defined, they nevertheless remain subject to infections and pain, and continue to carry body odors.

There is a fundamental difference between symptoms produced when nutoxins are leaving the body, and symptoms occurring because they have not. By analogy, if you clean your house by sweeping the dirt out the door, you will raise a lot of dust — but the house will be left clean, and you can repeat the process when needed. On the other hand, if your method is to sweep the dirt under the rug, sooner or later the place will become too dirty to live in no matter how often you "clean" it.

If you were standing down the street watching the first kind of housecleaning, you might see, along with the dust clouds, dog's hair, food scraps, bits of a broken glass, and a torn shoelace, emerging through doors and windows. You might even see an old chair or T.V. set tossed out. A similar situation holds for the human body. Nutoxins, like dust, may emerge at any one of the body's numerous "doors" or "windows" into the outside world — in other words, every point where body cells are in touch with the environment.

Although we usually think of our skin as the "outside" of our bodies, we do in fact also touch our environment through our mouth, ears, lungs, sinuses, stomach, intestines, vagina and elsewhere. At a cellular level, the interface between the "inside" and the "outside" of an adult human being is enormous. The total contact surface of an adult's intestines covers about 60 square feet. If each cell were scaled to the size of a Coke bottle, the area covered would be larger than Manhattan. The lungs with all their sub-structures would cover a city as well.

Normally, the body does not eliminate wastes equally over its entire "surface," but uses specific channels: primarily the bladder, intestines and bowel, and secondarily the skin and lungs. Normal elimination happens spontaneously and passes almost unnoticed. It is a natural function, and its mechanisms are inherent to us, the genetically determined product of millions of years of natural evolution.

But our normal cleansing *capacity* is also a product of evolution, and this is where problems arise in today's industrialized environment. When we are required to process and discharge types and amounts of toxins going far beyond those found in nature, our normal processes become overtaxed, or may no longer suffice at all. Then abnormal (non-usual) processes are forced into play. And these, when they become severe enough to be noticed, are what we call "symptoms."

When do symptoms mean that toxins are leaving the body? If we can identify these symptoms perhaps we can also have enough good sense to leave them alone.

The Symptoms of Detoxination

1. *There is a discharge of bodily matter carrying abnormal odors.*

The "matter" may be fluid, in the form of pus, sputum, a vaginal discharge or supurating wound, or it may be seemingly dry, in the form of dandruff, a rash, or flaking skin. If the only matter being discharged is the normally occurring urine and feces, detoxination is signified by the *presence* of *abnormal odors*.

Symptoms that are signs of detoxination are *useful* for the body, even if temporarily unpleasant. If they are unusual, it is because they constitute unusual methods of cleaning, needed when the ordinary ones are not up to the job. Such symptoms will spontaneously disappear once they have served their purpose (once no nutoxins are left to be flushed out). This means that the kinds of symptoms known to be *spontaneously self-terminating* should not be "treated." Do not shut doors and windows while house cleaning is in progress.

2. *The symptoms are spontaneously self-terminating.*

It is extremely important for the long-term integrity of the organism that detoxination symptoms be allowed to occur unmolested. Suppressing them with drugs may seemingly "cure" them in the short run, but the drugs will only add further toxins to the ones the symptoms were helping evacuate. Unless they are so severe as to endanger life, no prescription should be offered for detoxination symptoms other than raw, native food and fresh water. Limiting treatment to these things alone will in most cases spontaneously cause the symptoms to subside in short order.

In the case of chronic complaints — symptoms that terminate spontaneously, and then reappear the same way, or symptoms that ebb and flow — again, they reflect intoxination levels. The more rarely you bring muddy boots into the house, the more rarely and the less intensely will it have to be cleaned.

3. *The symptoms appear* (or their intensity increases) *when denatured foods or drinks are consumed,* and *disappear* (or decrease) *with natural, sense-selected nourishment.*

4. *There is fever or inflammation* in conjunction with the three preceding criteria.

When the fever occurs, it means that blood circulation through the body's tissues has increased dramatically because it was called for by the organism. In other words, the body *needs the increased irrigation.* Fever is a system-wide phenomenon, while inflammation, that serves the same purpose, is a similar one functioning locally.

Where fever or inflammation is occurring in association with at least one of the first three criteria, it should be construed as a toxin-related symptom and not be suppressed or "treated" unless it is unbearable or represents a danger to life. Fever that is not obviously associated with detoxination should, of course, be evaluated and treated medically (as should any other symptoms) with this proviso: if the physician is unaware of the etiological potency of foods, an attempt should be made to educate him, and failing that, to find a physician who is (aware, or . . . educable).

If you actually use (*do* and do not only *discuss*) the method of instinctive nutrition as explained in Part III, you will soon be able to recognize detoxination symptoms when they occur. If you avoid intoxinating yourself further at that time, you will prevent the symptoms from becoming severe and hasten their disappearance. And if you can avoid reverting to a high toxicity diet, you should soon find yourself in better health than you ever thought possible.

Chapter 11

A Black Hole
In (Medical) Space

Under Anopsological conditions, symptoms that meet the forego-
ing criteria will be understood by both patient and physician to
be health-*restoring.* Under so-called "normal" conditions, they will
usually be perceived as *destructive,* something to be "fought" and
repressed as quickly as possible. "Normal" denatured diets do,
in fact, so exacerbate macroscopic physiological and psychological signs (as a result of the underlying sub-microscopic and
microscopic chaos they produce) that symptoms may indeed easily become unbearable and even potentially lethal.

So it makes sense that in its ignorance of the profound effects
of food, the business of traditional allopathic medicine should
be to "treat" (eradicate) symptoms. It makes even more sense if
the assumption is made, as it generally is, that an *absence of patently
unpleasant symptoms = good health.* This assumption warrants

examining. By Anopsological standards, the "normal" (i.e., unnaturally fed) population in so-called "good health" is not in good health at all.

We should remember that the science (or art) of medicine is a *social* calling. It can only be based on the study of sickness and well-being in the society it evolved in. Its practitioners, as members of that society, share its beliefs. If the society at large makes no distinction between genetically natural and unnatural foods, medical practitioners are not likely to either. And historically, *no society on record has ever done so.* We know of no people on earth since the advent of agriculture that has ever had a diet devoid of denatured foods. So from their very beginnings until this day, medical theories, research, diagnoses, and treatments, have, without exception, been dealing with populations whose functioning was *not truly normal for humans.* It has been denatured by abnormal diets.

We were never able to recognize this before because no studies had ever been made of truly well-nourished people, who were eating foods to which they were genetically adapted, in kind and amount determined by their innate biochemical demands. These studies are now under way. They are providing a new frame of reference, and new standards for health and disease against which to compare the old. And they are radically changing our notions of what "normal" means for human beings. Some of them are discussed in the following chapters.

Because they call for a revision of many current assumptions in medicine, nutrition, and other related fields* these studies may not be welcome. Medicine has traditionally considered nutrition as all but irrelevant to pathology (an assumption shared by the chemical drugs industry, which is founded upon it).[1] It has good reasons to continue to do so, even in the face of contradictory evidence. For although medicine is defined as a "profession," it also qualifies as a *business.* The services it sells do not necessar-

---

* *These studies call for a reunion of psychiatry, biochemistry, dietetics, medical jurisprudence, etc.*

ily fill true needs. For it thrives, unfortunately, like many religions have done, on a mixture of *fear* and *hope*.

Usually, people are unwilling to pay for medical examinations and treatment unless they have something wrong with them (or believe they do), are afraid of it (and afraid it is going to get worse), and hope doctors and drugs will cure it. If they are not afraid, they'll try to take care of the problem themselves. If the physicians can offer no hope, they'll stop buying. The waiting rooms would be empty but for these two feelings.

Anopsology attenuates both. Most of the symptoms an instinctotherapy patient may experience will be unlikely to frighten him excessively because, for one thing, the symptoms will tend to be relatively mild, and for another, *he will better understand their meaning* — which in itself is an antidote to fear. Furthermore, physical pain subsides dramatically under Anopsotherapeutic conditions, and as the nervous system quiets down, anxiety disappears. At the same time, original nutrition heightens sensitivity, not only to smell and taste, but to body sensations in general, so the patient is able to experience his own spontaneous healing processes at work. He no longer needs "hope" that something outside himself will "do" a cure "to" him.

Confronted with the lessons of Anopsology, physicians may have to make some difficult choices. They may, as some already have, dismiss it out of hand with a demand for massive statistical data or unequivocal "proof" that the theory is "true" (not knowing or not admitting that only plausibility but no "proofs" exist for *any* medical hypothesis).[2] On the other hand, they may, as some have, study what has been learned, explore it themselves, and when appropriate, recommend it to patients. Anopsology is not patently antithetical to medicine, only to its abuse and misuse. Fortunately, some members of the medical profession do indeed practice the ethics they preach, and have dared advise their patients that "an apple a day keeps the doctor away" (on condition its smell and taste are attractive) — even though it might not have been the best thing for their wallets. No doubt there will be others who will do this in the future.

The idea of following a diet had always bothered me. I had never been interested in counting calories according to a prescription, grazing on plants or pecking grains. My wife was ill, but I would not have wanted her to follow any such method to cure herself.

Why was I so fascinated from the start with the instinctual selection of original foods? Why was I so dedicated to convincing my wife to apply it?

Here there were no contrived, restrictive theories. No mysterious hard-to-test treatments. No uncertain medicines with their perverse side-effects. No preparations at all were involved.

The only rule was: pleasure. *Smell and taste. The prescription is on the table in front of you, and you yourself are the doctor. All you have to do is reach out, smell, taste, choose . . . and eat.*

Antonin[3]

---

[1] The manufacturers of "food supplements" are vendors of *chemicals*, not of foods, so they are likely to share this sentiment.

[2] The absence of large-scale data does not in itself invalidate small-scale data.

[3] From "Orkoscopie," newsletter of the French National Anopsological Center.

Chapter 12

Food For Allergies

In order to understand how instinctive food therapy works, let us begin by looking at the bewildering problem of allergy, usually termed a "disorder." This suggests, if you suffer from it, that something is wrong with you. Something *is* wrong — but not with *you*.

The current medical model for allergies assumes that the organism has (for reasons unknown) become "hypersensitive" to some foreign substance (an allergen) to which it overreacts, and that further inputs of the allergen will further increase the organism's "sensitivity" and reactions, and so on indefinitely. It follows logically that attempts should therefore be made to 1) avoid the allergen, 2) decrease the sensitivity to it and/or 3) suppress reactions to it.

In point of fact, your organism is "sensitive" to ANY incoming substances whose antigenic marking is foreign. This is what triggers (or should trigger) the production of antibodies that will destroy the "alien" and eliminate it from your body. Therefore, to whatever degree (2) and/or (3) above are successful, they are to that degree dangerous for your long-term integrity. The reason is that "allergic" reactions are saying something important: they are announcing the fact that the allergens are toxic and therefore *dangerous*. Suppressing the reactions artificially may produce apparent (usually temporary) relief, but will result in the allergens *accumulating* within you — because you will no longer even feel a need to avoid them.

As we will see, however, what needs to be avoided is probably not what your reactions or test results show you to be allergic to. Once we light the fuse, are we then going to say the explosion was caused by the match? Allergens are detonators, but they are not the powder.

Allergic reactions are protective reactions. They are normal. Normally, they should occur wherever alien material touches the body's "surface." *Normally* they should be *confined to the sole site of the allergen's point of contact* (e.g., the nasal epithelium, the intestinal wall, etc.). And normally there the reactions should end, their number limited to the number of allergens. And that is the way it would happen, but for the *prior accumulation* in the body *of nutoxins whose structure is similar to the allergen*.

In other words: a person can only be "allergic" to molecular structures similar to the nutoxins he is already loaded with.

The nutoxins accumulated because the immune system either did not recognize them as foreign when they entered the body, did not respond with attempts to eliminate them, or did not succeed in doing so. When this has occurred — when the body is putting up with the presence of toxic material — the immune system is said to be in a state of TOLERANCE.

The reason the symptoms are called "allergy" in the first place is that they occurred in response to substances *that would normally be considered innocuous* — in contrast to recognized toxins. No one is said to be "allergic" to toadstools or bad oysters but if someone reacts strongly to strawberries (which are *not supposed to be toxic*), then he is said to be "allergic" to them. Persons who react strongly to bread, fried potatoes, and other foods, are by definition "abnormal" (i.e., they have a "food allergy") because bread, fried potatoes, and that other food are by definition "normal" foods for humans. In fact, they are not at all normal for our species, as we have pointed out.

After you have been eating instinctively for a time, you probably *will* have "allergic" reactions to bread (among other things) and it is not likely to surprise you (or worry you) at all. You won't find such reactions any more abnormal (i.e., "allergic") than your reactions to ammonia or cigar smoke.

It is important to understand that *an ordinarily useful substance may become toxic when ingested in excess.* Too much of a "good thing" = no longer such a good thing. Furthermore, any food that has been denatured to some extent will inevitably be toxic to a degree, since the human biochemistry is not prepared to correctly metabolize its altered molecular structure. The damage might be limited were there some way for the body to indicate when it had had all it could handle of that particular item. But our innate, alliesthetic (taste-change) response functions correctly only with foods in their original (native) state, not with denatured ones. And it does not function with mixtures of foods in any state — so by adding sugar to strawberries, we can trick our instinct into finding them good long after their taste would have turned us away, and come down with a rash or some other "allergic" reaction . . . to the *excess*, not to strawberries.

As another example: many babies have "allergic" reactions to cow's milk, which may include vomiting, diarrhea, rash, heavy sweating, watering of the eyes, or coughing up mucous (all of them detoxination symptoms). These responses are not perceived as the body's natural and spontaneous rejection of an unnatural food it cannot assimilate. Our culture believes so strongly that cow's milk is a good and necessary food for young humans, that if the two don't get along then something must be wrong with the baby rather than with the milk.

So the milk is forced on the baby, and in most cases, after a time, he will cease to react "allergically" to it. The parents will be relieved to see that he has overcome his "unnatural" reactions to this "natural" food. But what has really happened is that baby has given up. He has learned (it is an organic and immune-system "learning," not a rational one) that it is pointless to keep struggling to reject a substance whose ingestion he is powerless to prevent. If you can't fight 'em, join 'em — so his immune system becomes tolerant. He now puts up with the alien molecular input, which begins to accumulate within and between the cells of his body. These are not accumulations of inert bits and pieces like gravel, but of electro-dynamic fields, actively related to their surroundings. Like garbage on a golf course or static on the radio, they will "mess things up," causing the individual at best to just not feel too good, and at worst to become chronically or "incurably" ill. But since the more serious consequences may not appear for many years, the cause/effect relationship will probably not be suspected (particularly by physicians for whom nutritional factors seem irrelevant).

The baby who continues to react "allergically" to milk (until hopefully it is no longer fed to him) stands a better chance for life-long good health than one who tolerates it. For it is the mismetabolized accretions from denatured food that disrupts our organic harmony, which is in itself the most basic cause of disease.

Now suppose you suffer from an allergy. You wouldn't if your body weren't laden with accumulated nutoxins — your reaction to a few invasive allergens would be limited to those allergens alone. They would be minute, local reactions, hardly perceptible. But the gun is loaded. Like pent-up anger, you are full of pent-up foreign matter, and your body is cocked to discharge it. All you need is a trigger.

Let's say you're a bread-eater, a consumer of heat-processed chemical compounds of wheat (which was alien to humankind's native alimentary spectrum even before it was baked). At some point you undoubtedly did have some negative reactions to bread, but you failed to recognize them, so you continued to eat bread and eventually became tolerant of it. But as a result, your cells have become loaded with its mismetabolized residues.

Now it is summer, and a microscopic bit of chaff or pollen from wheat or other grasses comes into contact with a cell in your nasal epithelium. Normally, a secretion should occur at that site, to isolate and rinse away the pollen, and it does. But instead of limiting its response to a few actual bits of invasive pollen (dynamic electro-static fields, not inert), the body responds as well to the dynamic fields of similar "grasses-type" structure that came from your daily bread — which are still there, stuck in your cells. So instead of a minor, imperceptible secretion from a few cells alone, a chain reaction starts, and millions of cells begin to isolate and rinse away the foreign wheat-like material they had been putting up with. Out comes your handkerchief.

As long as you continue to eat bread, you will be prey to hay fever. The accumulation levels in your cells will vary, and so will your degree of tolerance, but when the equation is right for it, you will have a hay fever "attack." Why aren't you "allergic" to pollen when you *aren't* having an attack — even though pollen is almost constantly present in the atmosphere?

The answer is: *food.* Keep on eating bread, and within a short time you will have accumulated enough to set the stage for another massive "allergic" detoxination crisis.

It is unknown for an instinctively fed person to have an "allergic" reaction to pollen or to anything else. Once your organism has been cleaned out, once it is no longer permeated with debris, there is nothing there it needs to get rid of. It won't need to undertake a general house-cleaning when invaded by a few irritants at specific sites. Dust and smoke will still provoke coughing, watery eyes, a washing away of the irritant, *as they should.* But there the reactions will stop, because there is no reason for them to occur except locally.

If the symptoms of "allergy" vary greatly, it is probably because our diets include such a variety of unidentified poisons. An "allergic" reaction reflects an attempt to eliminate them. But toxins being ejected from the cells must pass through the bloodstream (which passes through the brain) on their way out. In so doing they can produce cramps, diarrhea, headaches, drowsiness, coughing, sneezing, uticaria, dizziness, palpitations, sweating, watering eyes, and altered emotional states, including unwarranted fears, anger and depression.

Instinctive nutrition provides an automatic cure for allergies of any kind, including "allergic" reactions to pollen, the sun, nylon or anything else. But artificially repressing the sensitivity or the reactions is not a *cure*, and in the long run it can be dangerous. If you eat the kinds and amounts of the foods you truly need and for which you were biochemically constructed, you will spontaneously rid yourself of the toxins gathered from your denatured nutritional past. For a time, your body will periodically smell strongly, as it discharges unuseable residues from the stews, soups, snacks and seasonings you consumed over the years — until you become perfectly odorless. At that point allergic reactions will have become impossible — along with inflammatory pain, fungus or bacterial infections and many other conditions.

Can these allegations be proved? You can do it yourself. Once you have learned to trust your instinct, they will become self-evident — at the cost of giving up a few traditions, habits and taboos, and by obeying the innate wisdom and felt demands of your own body, in preference to catalogued prescriptions designed to treat symptoms instead of their cause.

Chapter 13

Food and Cancer

Cancer cells are mutant cells that should normally be destroyed by the immunological system as soon as they appear. But the immune system is dozing, so to speak. It is already in a generalized *state of tolerance*; it has become passive. It has given up destroying not only pseudo-metabolites, but cancer cells as well.

Cancer cells might even be presumed to be feeding upon pseudo-metabolites (for they apparently fail to thrive in their absence). Their aberrant development might be thought of as a perfectly normal but unsuccessful attempt to adapt to aberrant food or other abnormal ("carcinogenic") input − a hypothesis fully as plausible as any other. In any case, no devilish "agent" *makes* cells cancerous; they become that way themselves.

While the relationship between *abnormal* food and cancer has yet to be correlated precisely, it is strongly supported (if we will look beyond our cooking pots to see it) by the results of a highly reputable study entitled, *"Nutrition and Its Relationship to Cancer,"* sponsored by the National Health Foundation:

Following up on leads advanced by epidemiologists, experimentalists have found that nutrition, in general, is related to the development of cancer in three ways: 1) Food additives or contaminants may act as carcinogens, cocarcinogens or both. 2) Nutrient deficiencies may lead to biochemical alterations that promote neoplastic processes. 3) Changes in the intake of selected macronutrients may produce metabolic and biochemical abnormalities, either directly or indirectly, which increase the risk for cancer.[1]

The study nowhere suggests that *denatured* nutrients might play a role in the etiology of cancer. The assumption is so widespread that cooked, canned, and frozen foods are "normal" for humans, that this omission should not be surprising. But the inference is suggested, for the study notes:

In Japan . . . an increasing trend has appeared associated with the progressive westernization of the Japanese dietary intake since 1945. This also provides some evidence that the dietary pattern, rather than the industrial activity, is one of the important factors in relation to causative mechanisms for these types of cancer: colon, breast, prostate.[2]

The study covered six types of cancer, including breast, large bowel, stomach, and head and neck, for which:

. . . the epidemiological evidence is overwhelming that nutritional factors have a major etiological role. Indeed, the epidemiological data on diet and nutrition in these four cancers provided the leads for metabolic and animal model studies that now fully support their epidemiological inspiration.[3]

The study states that for cancers of the pancreas and prostate, "the epidemiological evidence (for nutritional causative factors) is presently not overwhelming."

From the Anopsological viewpoint, there is no doubt whatsoever that denatured nutrients — or more specifically, their inevitable mis-metabolism — play a major role in the etiology of *any* type of cancer. We need only smell the patients. Every cancer patient ever examined under Anopsotherapeutic conditions carried highly unpleasant odors – often suggesting putrified milk products. More significantly yet: *as their tumors faded so did their body odors.*

We might think of a cancer as a campground supplied with whatever particular types of aberrant food and/or other conditions the cancer cells have adapted to. If the neoplasm (new growth) is incompletely removed by surgery (if all the campers are not destroyed – which usually implies the destruction of much of the surrounding landscape), the remaining cancer cells, now homeless, may locate elsewhere creating *metastases*, new colonies. Using indiscriminate chemical or radiation therapy that may or may not kill the survivors (but that will inevitably kill tremendous numbers of normal, healthy cells) is like flooding an entire city to put out fires in a few trashcans. A better solution would be to *starve* the cancer cells by providing nutrition suitable for normal cells only, which will also reactivate the immunological system against cancerous ones.

If food can cause cancer, might food not also cure it?

The following letter, written by a practicing physician, bears witness to the healing power of raw food selected by instinct. It was addressed to the French Social Security Administration to solicit Social Security coverage for patients in Instinctotherapy. (Reprinted by permission.)

Gentlemen,

I have had the opportunity through courses at the Paris Faculty of Medicine at Bobigny, to discover and employ a new therapeutic technique known as Anopsotherapy.

Over the past year I have been able to evaluate its remarkable results in illnesses of the greatest variety:

• In metabolic, particularly dyslipemic, illnesses, where the results were the total *normalization of biological values with no complimentary therapy, even in highly pathological cases. Regression of cardiovascular pathology was also noted: in angina, arteritis of lower members, and others (with clinical improvement in EKG, Doppler, etc.).*

• *In digestive pathology, in particular duodenal ulcer, and colitis even with a very long history.*

The most spectacular results concern the immunitary area:

• *In varied cases of allergies that were completely cured in a few weeks, including even cases with a long history.*

• *In Intrinsic asthma, which underwent rapid and major regression at the same time that the classic treatment was reduced and then halted (even in cortico-dependent cases). — In various chronic infections including genito-urinal, nose & throat, bronchial problems, etc.*

The most surprising results, however, although in limited number, were two auto-immune pathologies:

1. Rapidly evolving multiple sclerosis, with rapid loss of motor functions in the four members. Stabilized at first within a few weeks, I subsequently witnessed a total remission in the superior members, and a partial remission in the inferior members over a period of 10 months of Anopsological treatment.

2. In a case of myopathia: the illness ceased to evolve, and this was followed by slow improvement of the motor function over a period of seven months of Anopsological treatment.

In two cancers of the colon (seminomas), in men aged 49 and 36 respectively; the first with pleuro-pulmonary metastases, the second with pulmonary metastases producing compression of the superior vein cava:

Anopsotherapy was the only treatment used for the first patient (who refused chemotherapy). The pleural mass regressed almost entirely in less than three months. Regarding the metastatic images of the pulmonary parenchyma, they are currently undergoing a slow regression after 10 months of treatment. There was recovery of weight and physical activity in less than eight months.

The second case was taken over after previous chemical treatment that produced excessive alteration of the patient's general state. It was a case of a second relapse in five years with [chemotherapy].

Anopsotherapy produced a spectacular dissolving of the tumoral masses in less than six months. When he strayed from Anopsological nutrition, the patient had a relapse in August, 1984. After this regression, whose radiological evolution was rapid, the radiological images seem to have stabilized when the patient again took up correct Anopsological practice. The patient refused [chemotherapy].

In conclusion: over a period of a year I was able to evaluate the results of this technique in numerous cases of chronic pathology and in a few cases of severe pathology.

These results are of course insufficient for establishing a statistically representative study in terms of percentage of effectiveness, but they were sufficiently convergent to affirm that we are dealing with a major therapeutic technique.

One of the obstacles to studying a larger group comes obviously from patients' reluctance to undertake therapy at the Montrame Center since it is not covered by their Social Security insurance. Such coverage would not only facilitate medical progress, but it would also lead to economic savings.

In one year of practice I was able to observe a reduction in medical costs, and a very clear reduction in hospital costs and in days lost from work resulting from the use of this method. Furthermore, because the method is of a nutritional nature, it is compatible with any other therapy, whose effects it reinforces.
It is my hope that in the framework of the convergent interests, for once, between patients' physical health, and the Social Security System's financial health, you will examine the file on Anopsology.

(Signed) Jacques Fradin, M.D.
27 September 1984

[1] *"Nutrition and Its Relationship to Cancer,"* American Health Foundation, 1980, page 239.
[2] Ibid, page 240.
[3] Ibid, page 241.

Chapter 14

Food and Auto-Immune Disease

In the case of cancer, the immune system has fallen down on the job, and has failed to prevent the spread of abnormal, alien cells. In auto-immune disease, just the opposite has happened: the immune system has gone crazy, and is attacking "normal" cells. How can this have come about?

Normally, the immune system would attempt to destroy and eliminate only matter that is alien to it. It seems, therefore, that if normal cells are attacked, it must be because they have been *identified* as alien. And how could such mistaken identity occur?

Once we have understood that mis-metabolized residues from denatured or unnatural foods do, in fact, become "hung up" and *accumulate* in the body, then we can see how in some cases, the cells themselves (and not only the residues they contain) might become targets for destruction.

This is the picture shown by auto-immune patients in Instinctotherapy. Early in the process, as the immune system begins to reawaken and becomes increasingly intolerant of toxic residues in the body, odors begin to appear from unnatural foods eaten in the past. (In auto-immune cases, the odors almost invariably suggest putrid dairy products — which is often true in cancer cases as well.)

Next in Instinctotherapy, the patient's condition may worsen temporarily as his immune system becomes more vigorous and intolerant of alien introjects (for it has been identifying whole cells as alien, not just a part of their content). So the danger arises that the body could destroy its own toxin-laden cells massively enough to cause death. Therefore, *great care must be exercised in treating auto-immune disease to insure that detoxination proceeds at a slow pace.*

Fortunately, the patient can regulate his own detoxination quite simply. Instead of eating an initially "delicious" food until its taste turns "bad," he stops eating when the taste becomes merely "good." This means he is not ingesting as much of that particular food as his body was demanding — for use in driving out and replacing mismetabolites. So his self-dismantling processes, intentionally left short on fuel, are forced to slow down.

After some weeks or months, the danger of uncontrolled self-destruction passes (once the targeted cells have become sufficiently cleansed of pseudo-metabolites for the immune system to cease identifying them as "alien" — once the immune system has become more "sane"). When this happens, and immune responses become focussed on nutoxins contained in cells, but not on cells as-a-whole, regeneration can begin.

When it does, improvement may be irregular, in a sinusoidal "up" and "down" pattern. But as long as instinctive nutrition is strictly adhered to, no "down" should ever be worse than the one before it. This assumes, of course, that when therapy began, irreversible damage had not yet occurred — that the pathology had not reached a "point of no return." But even where the degenerative process can only be arrested but not reversed, patients are spared further deterioration.

Significantly, a number of auto-immune patients on the road to recovery have reported that worse-than-last-time relapses would occur if they strayed from proper instinctive practice — but *only* if and when they did so.

The following is reprinted from *Orkoscopie,* newsletter of the National Anopsological Center.

No, I must not keep silent. For all those who doubt, wait and hope, I must tell them! It is by means of these words that I am address-ing all those whom I do not know, so as to give them confidence and hope.

It was in March, 1983. A friend tells me about this farm not far from Toulouse where astonishing results are being obtained with all sorts of illnesses.

Suffering myself from an illness carrying the name of "Myelitis," a stylistic pirouette on the part of my doctors, who wished to spare me a verdict of Multiple Sclerosis, my friend incites me vivaciously to go to Les Berbaux. I am welcomed by Nicole Burger and a friendly group of people I don't know.

Before going any further, I must say that deep in my heart, I was not holding much hope, since I had already vainly tried natural and allopathic medicine (including corticotherapy). I told myself that this new therapy would also end up in failure. I might add that when I reached Les Berbaux, I was dependent on my wheel-chair, and was able to get around only with very great difficulty with English canes. After four years of vain efforts, I believed I was beyond recovery, and all I could hope for was to delay by daily struggle, the implacable evolution of my paralysis.

Nevertheless I listen attentively to Nicole Burger's explanations. Very quickly, and in spite of my initial qualms, I am seduced by the logic and the rigor of the reasoning. The meeting is therefore very positive and an appointment is made for the following week.

What a surprise I discover that in effect I am attracted by the smell of food for which I had no desire intellectually. Would I have ever dared eat 15 raw egg yolks in one sitting? And this passion lasts for several months before eggs suddenly became distasteful.

From elimination to elimination (read: "From one detoxination event to the next" — please refer to the chapter on "Nutritional Intoxination") *slowly my health improves: the trembling regresses during the first weeks, my general state is at a stable high, and I am less fatigued.*

Here it is the month of June, and I have three months of vacation ahead of me. Why shouldn't I spend them at Les Berbaux? In effect, these last months I was practicing Anopsology all alone, with no refrigerator, I was unbalanced. The biggest problem came from not having a wide enough choice of food, and I couldn't reach the taste-stop because I didn't have a large enough amount. Also because the products I could buy were not always original. During this period I had no improvement in my ability to walk (but no worsening either).

So for me the most reasonable answer was to be at Les Berbaux where the optimal conditions were brought together to insure a good result.

What a surprise when on July 18th I was able for the first time to walk 50 meters without a cane! Of course, my balance wasn't perfect, but what a reward all the same!

For a short time now I have been surprised to find that I am forgetting my inseparable crutches. It's like a game on a playing field in the house to try to find them! The day before yesterday I was able, for the first time in years, to drive my car like anyone else, pressing on the pedals with my feet like anyone else, without recourse to the special manual devices that I had had to have installed in order to be licensed to drive. What a joy to feel myself becoming normal again!

Some people who came to Les Berbaux recently for a seminar even asked me innocently: "But you, what are you here for?"

I couldn't help laughing, I who had seen myself condemned to a wheelchair for life! . . .

This will serve to conclude. I would so like to give back hope and confidence to those who will read this. For them too, an improvement and even a cure are possible. For that, the primary condition, it seems to me, is to practice Anopsotherapy seriously, without any errors, and with faith in our own bodies!

Of cource financial problems and psychological blockages can be obstacles, but are they really more important than good health?

Francoise

Chapter 15

Food and Diabetes

Diabetes is the name of a dysfunction of sugar metabolism that is not understood. It leads slowly to degeneration of the entire body, and normally never heals by itself. Medical treatment cannot cure it, only control it to some extent. The price of treatment is high, since the drugs (in particular, insulin) give rise to new symptoms, which cannot be successfully treated either. One of the most critical side-effects of the treatment is loss of sight. What is the diabetic to do?

The following can only give an indication of the potential value of instinctive nutrition in treating diabetes — for halting the progress of the disease, at least, if not curing it. Once again, it shows that *denatured food denatures the functioning of the person who eats it* — and points out a path that neither diabetics nor medical research can afford to neglect.

For every diabetic known to have tried it, instinctive nutrition rapidly reduced insulin dependency by at least 50% — and usually more. In theory at least, if this nutrition were adopted from the onset of diabetes, it might well enable new diabetics to avoid becoming dependent on insulin at all.

From a personal report addressed to Dr. Jean de Bonnefon in Paris. Reprinted by permission.

I have been diabetic for nearly 17 years, using three injections of insulin daily for a total of 40 units. I was able to reduce this dosage rapidly by a quarter and then by half. I did have an unpleasant period of detoxination, with glycemia over 2.50 g., but for the past 15 days my need for insulin has been only 10 units; my glycemia is often nearly normal, there is no longer any sugar in my urine, and acetone appears rarely or only as a trace.

Concerning my retinopathy, I had been seeing an ophthalmologist every three to six months, and at my last consultation I was told that "the inner eye is getting well." I was told to stop taking the two sorts of pills I had been using for seven years for blood circulation because they were no longer needed, and the next appointment has been set for a year from now.

I also had a necrosed thyroid nodule that appeared six months after beginning treatment for a hyperthyroid condition that started three years ago. From the last echograph it appeared that the necrosed tissues had all but completely disappeared!

Finally — I just feel good. I rapidly became much calmer and patient in my professional life. I saw my cellulite disappear, something I had never been able to get rid of. I have no more digestive problems, no more colitis, no more intestinal gas.

My diabetics specialist has witnessed these improvements, but says not enough time has passed. Clearly, the disappearance of the necrosed tissues of the nodule is unexplainable; in 400 similar cases he knows of, nothing similar was ever observed, even with hormone treatment. Nevertheless, he advised me to "not eat too much fruit." But I trust my instinct!

I will make an appointment three months from now to keep you up to date.

Genevieve

Chapter 16

Food and the Practice of Medicine: I

The following opinion, by a well-known French physician and medical writer, was written in support of Social Security health insurance coverage for patients in Anopsotherapy.

What I Think About Anopsology
by Jean de 'Bonnefon, M.D.

I. Unlike philosophical or naturopathic diets, all of which are *exclusion* diets based on an idea (e.g., vegetarianism, vegetalism, macrobiotics, etc.), Anopsology does not appear dangerous to me in that it allows for all foods except milk: glucides, lipids, animal or vegetable proteins, and even the use of as many as possible in all their natural variety. It is safe on condition that it be correctly applied, through the use of olfactory and gustatory instinct once they have been reawakened.

II. Anopsology is not medicine since it makes no use of diagnoses, chemical products or technical expedients. On the contrary, it counters alimentary artifice, which we are beginning to see is endangering our health and is a cause of disease.

It is not even a diet, since no dietary prescription exists. In effect it is the individual who chooses. It is his body that does so, not his mind. And his body probably knows better than any computer what it needs, and what is most useful in an ongoing and specific way.

Anopsology is in no way contrary to, or incompatible with medicine. The usefulness and necessity of medicine is preserved in fighting symptoms and illnesses, while Anopsology consolidates the terrain by way of its nourishment.

In my view, Anopsology can only reinforce tolerance to, and the effectiveness of, chemical medicine.

Medicine and Anopsology are therefore complementary. And this is true even in cases of severe illness, where it is appropriate to employ as many weapons as possible.

III. In practical terms, insofar as I have been able to see and experiment, Anopsology is surprisingly effective as concerns the improvement of well persons, and a return to health for sick ones.

IV. On theoretical grounds, Anopsology addresses three essential questions:

1. the disturbing problem of the accelerating denaturation of our food.

2. the problem of the role of our alimentary instinct, completely ignored by our teaching hospitals.

3. the question of our genetic and enzymatic adaptation to our nutrition.

This theory even makes it possible to establish a connection between these sciences.

In resume, this method of nutrition, on condition that it is correctly applied, is the best dietetic approach I know of, and I feel that its application in the form of an intensive cure can be extremely useful for our health.

> – Jean Devernois de Bonnefon, M.D.
> Former Clinic Chief, Salpetrière Hospital, Paris
> Medical Expert at the Paris Court of Appeals
> 13 July 1984

Food and the Practice of Medicine: II

> *Dr. Catherine Aimelet was consulting physician at the experimental Instinctotherapy Center near Paris through 1984 and 1985. As a physician, her role was mostly advisory, since few prescriptions were called for once patients had begun the therapeutic process. As the body receives the nutrients it can metabolize correctly, it can and does eliminate the mismetabolites from denatured foods eaten previously. Detoxination "crises" do occur, however, and only a trained physician who understands what is involved, can tell whether there is any danger for the patient. The following is an abridgement of a report she prepared for other doctors investigating the therapy.*

This is a general report on patients I have examined who were using Instinctive Nutrition therapeutically. I am including a few characteristic cases of severe pathology who benefited from this alimentary reeducation (and re-provisioning, as it were).

I am also including a partial list of dysfunctional or "minor" complaints that benefited. In these cases patients were able to reduce or in most instances entirely halt medication, and avoid additional examinations and analyses, hospitalization, etc. There were many cases of this type, and they will be included in our statistical studies (that will take a great deal more time than we have had to date).

It was my duty at the Center to follow patients who were staying for at least two or three weeks or longer, as well as collect biological and clinical data on them in cooperation with their personal physician. I can state that Anopsotherapy was unquestionably beneficial in the following types of conditions:

 — Auto-immune pathology
 — Chronic and repetitive dermatoses
 — Biermer's anemia
 — Hemophilia (Deficiency of factor VII)
 — Acute infectious pathology
 — Neoplastic pathologies

It goes without saying that during the course of instinctive nutrition therapy, medical treatment was maintained if required.

Other conditions that responded well to this method included:

 — Migraine headaches
 — Obesity and overweight problems
 — Rheumatism
 — Tobacco addiction
 — Dyspeptic problems
 — Constipation and diarrhea
 — Gastritis and ulcer of the duodenum
 — Allergies
 — Chronic children's ear, nose and throat infections
 — Chronic and repetitive vomiting in pregnant women
 — Cardio-vascular problems:
     — High Cholesterol levels
     — Tachycardia
     — Arteritis
     — Coronary pathology
     — Veinous insufficiency
 — Anxiety and depression
 — Insomnia
 — Genito-urinary infections

Following are several case histories that illustrate the above.

* * *

ALAIN: Born: 1940

1973 – Hepatitic colic
1974 – Cholecystectomy
1976 – Nephritic colic
1978 – Prostatitis with complications
1981 – Proteineuria
1982 – Viral Hepatitis, asthma, asthenia – unable to work. By October, 1982: general deterioration of health. Biopsy showed chronic active hepatitis evolving toward cirrhosis of liver. 1983: Worsening general state. No treatment considered valid.

Began Anopsotherapy in May, 1984. Weight: 52 Kg.
General state improved rapidly. By December had normal transaminase. By May, 1985: very good state of health. Began working full time in September, 1985.

In summary: Auto-immune disease with liver and kidneys affected in process of healing. Patient's health excellent.

* * *

VINCENT: Age 2 1/2 in April, 1985.

The child had been fed original foods by instinct from the age of one year (with occasional small amounts of cooked foods). In April, 1985 the child falls into a fireplace, burning the palms of both hands to the 3rd degree. Is taken to emergency burn clinic at hospital. Proposed treatment includes: hospitalization, antibiotics, sterile chamber, bathing of wounds. Doctors foresee ablation of necrosed tissues and probable amputation of the more severely burned right hand. Mother refuses and takes child to Anopsotherapy center.

Between 1st and 5th day: serum drains continuously from burned areas, but the child begins to move his fingers and has *no complaints of pain.*

Between 6th and 10th day: noticeable improvement, with child fully using his hands, which are visibly healing.

By the 30th day: no visible trace of burn, no scars, no sequels.

* * *

CELINE: Born: 1970

At age 1 month diagnosed as hemophilia (deficiency of factor VII). 1970 to 1977: multiple hemorrhages (3 per week average). Treated with PPSB or PFC + transfusions. 1977: EEG perturbed. Salmonellas. Chronic anemia. "Pre-autistic" state, anorexic.

Began Instinctotherapy in 1979 at age 7.

Results: In six months: Improved general health. Rapid improvement of blood chemistry. Progressive reduction of spontaneous hemorrhaging, infrequent need for treatment.

By the end of one year: satisfactory body growth. Normal biological values, coagulation normal, bone calcification normal. To date: Normal intellectual development, does well in school, normally socialized, practices sports. Continues to eat instinctively.

* * *

ROSELINE: Age 61

Rheumatoid arthritis beginning in 1982, wrists affected. Latex Waller Rose test highly positive. Increasing stiffness, redness, pain and inflammation spreading to knees, shoulders and elbows. Anti-inflammatory treatment beginning in 1984 was halted because of gastro-intestinal side-effects. Turned to naturopathy, with diet of eggs, vegetables, limited fruit and rice, for nine months. Then reverted to "normal" diet for two months which caused symptoms to "explode," paralyzing her.

Began Anopsotherapy in May 1985, at home, with fruits and vegetables. By third day had high fever and articulations were blocked (there was no elimination of toxins). When she began correct practice at the Center, all pain was gone in three weeks.

During the fourth month detoxination began seriously with skin infections (abcesses) on fingers, hands, top of wrists and at base of spine. Was attracted almost exclusively to overripe fruits and spoiling fish during this period which lasted a month. Then skin infections subsided and healed overnight, and she recovered movement of articulations (with minor stiffness remaining occasionally). Extremely active and in good health: now easily hikes eight kilometers or more. In conclusion: Rheumatoid arthritis regressed almost completely in nine months.

Chapter 17

Food for Tension and Stress

It may not be an exaggeration to suggest that even wars may be caused by denatured food. Once you have been eating instinctively for a few weeks you will understand why. You will probably say, "I used to be a buzz-bomb!" When your body has become sufficiently cleansed of some of its load of accumulated nutoxins, then without drama or fanfare, inner peace will come into being — no tranquilizers required. Your mind will become quiet, your ideas stop racing. And you will then (but only then and not before) become aware of what unnatural food was doing to you.

The neurological mechanisms involved have never been explored, for the good reason that their existence was never suspected. Medical research to date has assumed that denatured foods were "normal" for humans, and so has remained unaware of the effects of *truly* normal (for humans) food. But you will be able to experience them yourself. If you later revert to a dinner of melted cheese on whole-wheat toast and soup, and discover that shortly thereafter you have become "unexplainably" anxious, tense and stressed, it will be unexplainable no longer.

Let us use a model to try to visualize what is happening.

The neurons, or nerve cells of the body, communicate with one another through "synapses" that function like junction boxes, collecting signals from incoming neurons and passing them on to others. The synapse will "fire" (i.e., pass an impulse "downstream" to the next cell in the circuit) only if enough "upstream" (incoming) pulses are present to produce a charge powerful enough to set it off. The synapses have minimal firing thresholds that are modified by drugs. Tranquilizers raise them, so that more input is needed for output to be produced. Stimulants have the opposite effect.

Thanks to observations of and by instinctively fed people, we now have a standard of comparison that leads us to infer, among other things, that abnormal food either causes so-called "normal" thresholds to be abnormally low, or creates an abnormally high level of internal nervous stimulation. The body enters a state of self-reflexive positive feedback, leading to organic frenzy. If you have ever observed a desperately hungry baby you will easily see what this means:

When baby is hungry, he begins to cry, and if not fed, his crying becomes louder and more insistent until his entire body is involved: his tension is all-encompassing, and will continue to increase until either 1) he is picked up and fed, or 2) he "gives up" — becomes exhausted and falls asleep. Baby's demands become so desperate that it would appear that he was in terrible pain and even starving to death — which is, in fact, just how he feels. This has been reported by patients in Primal Therapy who relived crib starvation (that occurred when, as babies, they were fed according to a fixed schedule rather than according to their needs), and expressed their early feelings in exactly those terms.[1]

When the starving baby is finally given the breast, he will at first nurse desperately, slowing down progressively until, at the end of his meal, he will suddenly stop nursing entirely and (as though with a sigh of relief), go limp (and probably fall asleep).[2]

As adults, we can no longer fully express ourselves the way babies do, but the lower brain structures that mediated our behaviors when we were born are still on the job. We are taught self-control from an early age — taught not to express or heed our hunger when it becomes intense. But even though we may have become unable to experience or show it directly, when we become hungry for the nutrients we need, the hunger will mobilize our nervous system just like a baby's, giving rise to the same sort of frenzy and pain it did earlier. Even though we may not scream and cry out our need, the hunger affects us *as a whole*, body and "mind" and everything else.

The electrical, neuronal stimulations of this organic, every-cell-involved pain is one thing that keeps a person keyed up, nervous, tense, stressed, anxious, angry, distressed and even clinically insane in some cases. The other of course, is the biochemical chaos produced by molecules never encountered in nature, which entered our bodies by way of our denatured foods.

> *Our brain is no different from the rest of our body. In fact, the brain is the body's most chemically sensitive organ. Starved for the right nutrients, or "gummed up" by toxic pollutants, the brain can and does go haywire...sugar starvation, vitamin deficiencies, lead pollution and food allergies can convert a normal brain into a criminal mind.*[3]

Short of creating a "criminal mind," it is clear that abnormal nutrition leads to abnormal behaviors of many sorts. Could even such psychological distortions as sexual perversion have unnatural food at their root? If cats (who suffer none of humankind's frequently aberrant psycho-social conditioning) can become perverted thanks to food, why not us?

> *Cats fed cooked meat show much more irritability. Some females are even dangerous to handle and three are named Tiger, Cobra*

and Rattlesnake because of their proclivity for biting and scratching. The males, on the other hand, are more docile, often to the point of being unaggressive and their sex interest is slack or perverted. In essence, there is evidence of a role reversal with the female cats becoming the aggressors and the male cats becoming passive as well as evidence of increasing abnormal activities between the same sexes. Such sexual behaviors are not observed among the raw food cats. [4]

Most people have food preferences, and where instinct is not at work (as it cannot be with denatured foods) our predilections will run not to what we *need* (since denatured diets rarely if ever provide it) but rather to the foods that will narcotize our pain. Foods or alcohol with a high sugar content at least provide a quick glucose "fix" against the suffering of hypoglycemia. Stimulants such as coffee and tea fortify our higher-brain repressive capacities that enable us to avoid the experience of distress (but since they are usually sweetened, they also raise our blood glucose levels). Many foods in our "normal" diets temporarily tranquilize us, while failing to provide the nutritional equilibrium that would relieve us. (Food supplements are unable to provide this correctly either.) Once proper nutritional balance has been established by instinct, then the pain of nutritional deprivation disappears – and with it, the need for tranquilizers of *any* sort.

For these reasons, it is not uncommon with instinctual nutrition to see a heavy smoker quit completely within only two or three days, or an alcoholic give up the bottle literally overnight. People with a "sweet tooth," many of them obese from the accumulations of unuseable cooked sugars, stop craving sweets. In fact, "craving" of almost any sort will subside because when the cells of the body are not lacking anything, there is no cause for them to crave anything. Interestingly, not only compulsive eating, but compulsive behavior of every sort subsides dramatically.

Two classes of denatured (and in this case, *unnatural*) food seem to contribute most severely to creating "stress." The first is *cereals*, the second, *milk* (and milk products). For millions of years, neither was on the human menu; they are recent innovations.

Most books on nutrition proclaim that whole-wheat bread is better food than white-flour bread, since it contains minerals and vitamins that refined flour has lost. But it also contains molecular structures of much greater complexity, which cooking transforms into chemical compounds of greater complexity that raise even more havoc with our nervous systems than refined wheat does. If you have been eating grains, particularly *whole* grains, you will probably notice almost at once when you give them up that you are less keyed up.

The same goes for milk, food for cows. It does not do nice things to humans.

> *In some situations, removing milk from the diet can result in dramatic improvements in behavior, especially in hyperactive children. In four out of five children, aged six to 15, found to be sensitive to milk, all reported "markedly positive" improvement when milk was completely eliminated from the diet.*[5]

The author of these lines had himself done a study of juvenile offenders that showed them to be drinking, on the average, more than twice as much milk as a comparison group of non-offenders. But he, like most of the population, holds the culturally inculcated assumption that cow's milk just *has* to be good for humans. He says: "Of course milk should still be considered a nutritious source of protein for children" — before going on to report a study conducted by the San Luis Obispo (California) county Probation Department:

> *Nearly 90 percent of the offenders had a symptom history associated with milk intolerance or allergy. Further examination and biochemical testing revealed 80 percent had evidence of milk allergy.*[6]

You should by now be getting the picture. To prevent or cure upset stomach, anger, tenseness, asthma, insomnia, restlessness, anxiety, depression, impatience, confusion, hostility and similar discomforts, you have to eat right.

In the next section we will explain how to do it.

[1] Please refer to the writings of Arthur Janov (see bibliography at the end of this volume).

[2] It should be pointed out that babies fed original foods in addition to their mother's milk do not demonstrate this sort of desperation.

[3] Michel Lesser, M.D., in his introduction to *Diet, Crime and Delinquency* by Alexander Schauss, Parker House, Berkeley, 1984.

[4] Francis M. Pottenger, Jr., *Pottenger's Cats*, op. cit. Please see Chapter 5 for a discussion of Pottenger's nutrition experiments.

[5] Alexander Schauss, *Diet, Crime and Delinquency,* Parker House, Berkeley, 1984.

[6] Please see Chapter 12 for a discussion of the meaning of "allergy."

PART III
DOING IT YOURSELF

Chapter 18

Another Way of Looking at Food

When the family sat down to dinner, each had a plate in front of them that looked like this:

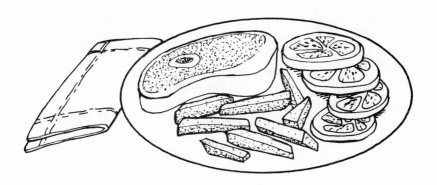

Prayers were said, and then Danny, age ten, dug in at high speed. Within minutes his plate looked like this:

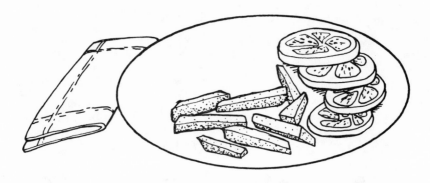

Then like this:

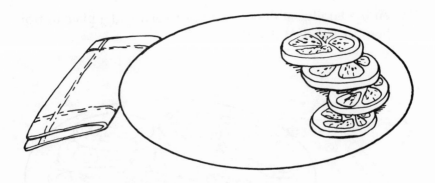

At this point Danny stopped eating. After a while, his father pointed to the items remaining and said, "Aren't you going to eat that?"

"I don't like tomatoes," said Danny.

"That's fine," said his father, "but what about *that?*" and pointed again.

"I don't like tomatoes!" screamed Danny.

"I heard you," said his father, "you don't like tomatoes." And he pointed at the round red slices remaining on the plate. "But what about *that?*"

Danny sat silent, perplexed. After a few minutes he timidly cut off a small piece of what was left on his plate and gingerly tasted it, chewing carefully. Hesitating, he cut off another . . . then another, until shortly his plate looked like this:[1]

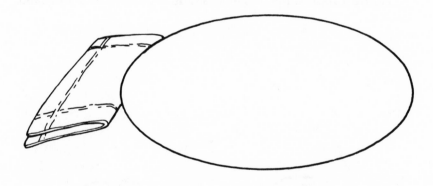

Although this story involves cooked foods, that aspect of it is irrelevant. It is the *mechanism* that counts. Had Danny's father not insisted that Danny's prejudgment could be mistaken, Danny might have grown up "not liking tomatoes" once and for all. A lot of people say they don't like one food or another — and won't even try them, for that reason. It seems perfectly reasonable, for why should someone force himself to eat something he *knows* he doesn't like . . . or even taste something he's *sure* he won't like?

Let's look at what is involved.

Let us imagine that at some point during Danny's early childhood, in 1956 let us say, he was offered a tomato that he tasted and didn't like. We'll call it "T1". If it was a raw tomato, unseasoned, in its original state, his biochemistry was causing him to dislike it because he didn't need it. However, his mother might have insisted he eat it, on the theory that tomatoes are healthy foods, always and everywhere "good for you." (Subjected often enough to this kind of reasoning, Danny might even come to the conclusion that only bad-tasting foods were "good for him," adopting as an unconscious nutritional credo: "the worse it is, the better it is".)

Figure 1 represents this evil-tasting tomato that day in 1956.

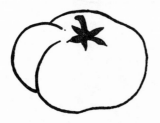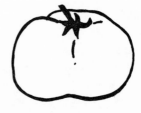

Figure 1   Figure 2

Some years later – and at various times over the years – Danny may attend a dinner party where he is offered a tomato. One of these tomatoes, "T2", in 1986 let us say, is represented in Figure 2. Danny will eat everything else, but he will not touch the tomato. If you ask him "Why not?", his reply will be, "Because I don't like tomatoes."

"But you haven't even tried it!" you might say, and Danny would answer, "I don't need to!"

From his first bad experience with a tomato – just one may have been enough – Danny created a generalization about them. Tomato 1 and tomato 2 look alike: their size, color, shape, etc., are almost the same. So Danny assumes they must *taste* the same. He is unaware that original foods *never* taste the same. Cooked foods usually do – but original foods vary in taste from one item to another of the same variety, and from one bite to another of the same item.

Furthermore – and here lies an insidious trap – T1 and T2 carry the same *name*. The very same label "Tomato" applies to both events, even though they are distant by 30 years. But in Danny's mind, it is perfectly rational to avoid anything that carries that name, because logically, for him, they are "the same thing."

For those of us who find ourselves trapped like Danny, it might be rewarding, at least occasionally, to *smell* and *taste* a food we may not previously have liked, before we declare it *non grata*. There is just no way to tell from its name what something will taste like at a given moment.

> The only person I really trust is my tailor. He takes my measure-
> ments every time I see him.
>
> George Bernard Shaw

Generalizations about foods, in whatever terms they are cast, are representations only; they are never the foods themselves. Reference tables abound listing the "contents" of herring, beef-steak, endives, peaches, almonds, and so on in terms of calories, fats, vitamins, minerals and other "components." They take no account of the differences between a greenhouse tomato in December and a vine-ripened one in August. They take no account of what nourished, or failed to nourish, the particular food we are eating (that our taste buds do take account of). Any two sardines may appear to be "the same" when judged by our higher brain structures, our non-sensing "mind" that understands lists of "ingredients." For our lower brain structures (that "make *sense*" but do not make "ideas"), each sardine is different from every other.

> *[Dietary calculations] seldom agree closely . . . We studied the vitamin content of meals already prepared to eat in homes. We weighed and calculated the nutrient content in each meal item using food tables, and compared the calculated amounts with the analysis amounts. In most cases the calculated value exceeded the analyzed value by 5 to 30 percent . . . More recently we conducted a study of dinner meals with the same results. The ascorbic acid content of the prepared meals by analysis was about 60 percent of the calculated value, the fat content was about 70 percent of the calculated value, etc . . .* [2]

The way we humans evaluate and process food biochemically in our bodies has thus far been studied more assiduously in laboratories than out in the real world we live in. Much has been learned about oxydants, hormones, fibers, amino acids, etc., and new biochemical entities, and new types of old ones, are turning up daily. So much information has been accumulated, in fact, including so much that is seemingly contradictory, that by now we can hardly even use it without some kind of nutritional philosophy as a guide. The logic of Anopson might qualify as a "philosophy" too — except that the mechanisms of genetic adaptation to foods developed long before those of brains fit for "thought." For several billion years, they have served as the basic nutritional guidance for every animal species on earth.

Eating by instinct is the simplest way there is. We need only to *trust our own nature and that of our foods.* Infants and children will do so spontaneously if allowed to. Adults, educated in ways aimed at developing "mind," may need to put forth an effort to *unlearn* what they "know," to make a place for sensations and feelings. We may stumble at first, and perhaps make mistakes. But merely starting gives confidence, and leads ultimately (and in a surprisingly short time) to a degree of satisfaction in being alive, that dead foods and prescribed ways of eating them simply cannot provide.

With this orientation in mind, let us explore the practice of instinctive nutrition.

---

[1] *No one ever told this story better than O. R. Bontrager of the University of Arizona at Tempe, with whom it originated.*

[2] Harris, R. S. (moderator) Panel Discussion: *Food composition and availability of nutrients in foods,* American Journal of Clinical Nutrition, Vol. 11, No. 5, Nov., 1962.

Chapter 19

Eating by Instinct

Human Foods

Anopsological, or instinctive, nutrition makes use only of foods that are "natural" *for humans*. In Chapter 3 we defined a "natural" food as one that was part of man's *native alimentary spectrum*, and that was in its *original state as found in nature*. In order to decide which foods were native to men, we proceeded by exclusion: we qualified as "unnatural" any foods that could not be consumed without the use of some artifice, or that had been denatured by thermal, chemical, mechanical or other means.

On this basis, we came to the conclusion that two types of foods found in nature were not native to men: cereal grains, and milk from non-human species, such as cows or goats. We reasoned that men could not have become adapted to them, because through millions of years of genetic evolution, they never ate them.

For this reason, Anopsological practice excludes all dairy products, whether raw or pasteurized (even though Pottenger's experiments showed that cats did well on raw milk). In nature, milk serves as a food for the new-born of a species, never as a beverage for the adults; and the milk of a given species is never consumed by another one. Significantly, animal milk in any form provides no alliesthetic protection for humans: its taste will not change to signal that the drinker has consumed all he needs. This alone signifies that milk, even raw — along with cheese, butter, and yoghurt, is not a native human food.

By raising cattle, man may have succeeded in producing a "natural" *artificial* food analogous to dwarf pigs or seedless grapes. Perhaps raw milk can, in fact, safely and usefully be consumed as a food, even though it produces no alliesthetic protection. Domestication, and artificial breeding, might account for the lack of a taste-change. Wild vegetables and fruits provoke strong taste transitions compared to their cultivated cousins, and meat from wild animals tastes stronger — and its taste changes more sharply — than domesticated meat. Would milk from wild cattle produce a taste-change to protect against toxic overload? We will never know because genetically wild cattle are extinct. The best we can do perhaps is to ask: does raw milk from wild reindeer or llamas, for instance, appeal to humans and change taste when they have had enough? If so, the absence of an alliesthetic response in raw milk would be due to selective breeding.

Cereals are another special case, and the argument that they "contain" carbohydrate, vitamins, and minerals, needed in human nutrition, does not alone justify eating them. Similar nutrients can be found in the seeds of practically any of the grasses or other plants, as well as in the plants themselves.

A particular problem arises here because cereal grains are *seeds*. In this respect they resemble sunflower seeds, peas, beans or nuts: they are the kernels from which new plants or trees will spring under proper conditions. But seeds, once they have matured and until they have germinated, are biochemically dormant: they contain enzyme inhibitors that protect them from decomposing like leaves or stalks would, long enough to find a niche in the soil, to become soaked through with moisture and germinate.

Once they have germinated, the enzyme inhibitors become inactive, and the seeds are "alive" again. And at this point, like any other food native to humans, they produce an odor and taste that may be appealing, and they can be eaten to satiety. They also become digestible with no need for cooking, precisely because their enzymes are not inhibited. This holds true for cereal grains as well as for other seeds, with one exception: *hybridized wheat* (and it is practically impossible to find any other kind). Germinated wheat will taste delicious to practically everyone *whether he needs it or not*. And *it will never stop tasting good*. In other words, artificial selection over thousands of years has biochemically modified wheat to the point where its structure today is no longer keyed to our genetic alimentary programming. It will no longer trigger a taste-change when satiety has been reached.

> In germinated tree nuts and cereal grains we can find all of the
> protein, carbohydrate, fat and calories we will ever need. The world
> is looking for someone to put these items on the market in a palata-
> ble form, untouched by heat and free from enzyme inhibitors.'

We might add that the world is looking for someone to culti-
vate wild wheat without "improving" it. Commercial wheat will not produce a taste-change for chickens any more than it does for humans. They will gorge themselves on it to the exclusion of other foods, often becoming ill. It is not used for raising foul to Anopsological standards, nor for cattle or other animals.

Aside from these exceptions, parts of practically any plant or animal found in nature can be eaten in their native state by human beings without ill effect, on the condition that their smell and taste are attractive. This includes herbs as well as reptiles and insects. The latter two are excluded from the discussion that follows because they are not thought of as "food" at all in most western societies (although iguanas, snakes, and eels, are consumed in many parts of the world, and insects as well, though more rarely).

For the purpose of this discussion, and for organizing instinctive meals, we will classify foods into groups. This system of classification is arbitrary to a degree and subject to revision; it is only a tool, not a "truth."

Food Groups

1a. Land animals (including chicken and bird eggs)

1b. Sea animals (including fish and turtle eggs)

2.   Fruits

3.   Vegetables (including roots and tubers)

4a. Nuts

4b. Seeds and legumes

5.   Honeys

In serving and eating meals, items from each group comprise a "course" that should be finished before moving on to the next one. We will explain this in detail in a moment.

Some of the foods in these groups that are often (although not always or everywhere) available on the commercial market are listed at the end of this chapter. They will be discussed individually in the following chapters.

Instinctive Meals

How Many Meals? Far in the distant past, our predecessors no doubt ate when they were hungry, or whenever they managed to find food, without waiting for a particular time of day, every day. We, however, usually follow a schedule such as Breakfast,

Lunch and Dinner. Instinctive eating works well in this frame-work, so there is no reason to give it up. In therapeutic practice, only two meals are served daily: lunch at noon and dinner at 7:00 p.m. This also works well. There is no need to establish an immutable rule; appetite is an excellent guide — and its appear-ance, in fact, is related to established habit patterns and biorhythms that should be respected. Compulsive nibblers and others who eat irregularly might do well to adopt a regular eat-ing pattern if they wish to obtain good results with instinctive nutrition.

How much food at each meal? There is little doubt that long ago in the wild, men gave little consideration to how much they intended to eat. Most of us today, however, do so almost uncons-ciously. The kinds and amounts of food served at different meals vary considerably in different cultures, and reflect our expecta-tions at different times of the day. A Continental breakfast will generally consist of little more than coffee and rolls, while a typical American breakfast might include eggs, sausage, and pancakes. Spaniards prefer to eat heavily at noon and lightly in the eve-ning, while the American pattern is just the opposite. Each of us will be influenced by his own customs, and fortunately, Instinc-tive Nutrition requires no hard and fast rules. Practical constraints will impose their own rules: for someone who has only half an hour for lunch, lunch will have to amount to little more than a snack. But insofar as one has a choice, the best pattern to follow is the one that provides *the most satisfaction*.

Organizing Meals

Breakfast. Most instinctive eaters are not hungry in the morn-ing. Once their metabolic homeostasis has reestablished itself, they have little need for an early morning catapult launch into the world with tea, coffee and "fast" carbohydrates as propel-lants. The body's nighttime eliminatory processes are still at work in the morning, and the body's own schedule need not defer to a clock saying "it's time" for breakfast. If a person is *actually hungry*, of course, he should eat, or drink water if he's thirsty. But breakfast every morning is no more a biological imperative than fish every Friday.

If the beginning student of instinctive nutrition will do with little breakfast or none at all for a few days, he will probably soon discover he doesn't miss it. At first, however, he is likely to be quite hungry by lunch time (which can be earlier than usual). In the beginning, there is a benefit to feeling very hungry instead of only mildly so: it sharpens the senses of smell and taste. They are still relatively blunted, desensitized by mismetabolized residues from a denatured-foods past.

The Anopsological approach to eating stands in sharp contrast to many of our normal habits, which many people may not wish to give up. We hope they understand that these comments are guidelines, not rules, Instinctive nutrition is not a closed dietary system, not a religion. It can be followed *in part*, and to any extent that it is used, still be beneficial to a degree.

If a person wants to preserve some of his long-standing nutritional habits — his morning coffee, for instance (preferably sweetened with honey rather than refined sugar or a chemical sweetener) — he may, with care, be able to do so with only minimal ill effect. But the less denatured food he consumes, the more his senses will awaken to guide him, the better will his health be, the more effective his organic self-repair. He need not fear the crooked path, for only by experimenting will he discover how foods, both natural and denatured, actually do affect him. He can test the method — just as he would test a food before eating it — and use as much or as little as suits him.

If he is hungry in the morning, he might try eating fresh fruit. Some honey might fit the bill as well. He might avoid juice because juice, even fresh, will not trigger a taste-change message to prevent toxic excess. He should certainly avoid cheese blintzes.

Lunch. Lunch may be a one-, two- or three-course meal of the following:

1st course — Group 2: fruits

2nd course — Group 4a: nuts

3rd course — Group 5: honeys

Only these food groups are usually eaten at lunchtime. However, if a person finds nothing among them to attract him, he should by all means test foods from other groups, starting with vegetables.

Occasionally a person may be in a metabolic readjustment phase, with such a pressing need for one kind of food only, that no others are appealing. He may find, for example, that *only* mussels appeal to him, or *only* asparagus. He should obey his senses, and eat that food exclusively until others again become appealing, perhaps a day or two later.

If a person finds nothing that really attracts him, it might also be that he's not really hungry, but is telling himself he *ought* to eat because it's lunchtime. Cultural conditioning by-the-clock is so widespread that some people may force themselves to have a meal "at mealtime" even when they're not hungry, or eat because they're afraid they *might* be hungry later on unless they do. A lack of appetite at noon does not necessarily forebode pangs of famine by mid-afternoon, however.

Courses are eaten *in sequence,* one after the other. The fruit course might consist, for example, of an assortment of bananas, pineapples, watermelon, oranges, grapefruit, grapes and strawberries. The greater the variety the better — but most people will be limited by availability and prices in the stores.

Each fruit should be smelled in turn *before beginning to eat any of them* (some fruit may require that the skin be scratched to bring forth a smell). Whichever fruit smells most appealing is the one to eat, and it should be eaten *until the taste changes from good to bad.* This may happen after the third peach or other fruit, or after the tenth. There is no way to predict how much of a particular fruit a person may consume. When the taste goes bad, when the eater has had all he *wants,* it means *his body has had all it needs.*

Anopsological meals do not include drinks. Fruit contains so much fluid that it is rare for anyone to need water in addition. Furthermore, water consumed during the course of a meal will dilute gastric juices and reduce digestive efficiency. When consumed alongside fruit, it is likely to produce fermentation: gas, and bloating.

After the taste of the first fruit has gone bad, a second may be selected, again by smell. Again, it should be eaten until the taste goes bad. This may happen almost at once, it may happen after the third or fourth fruit, or it may not happen at all before the eater becomes "full." For the beginner, however, whose palate is not yet resensitized, feeling "full" may be an illusion. If someone stops eating a fruit on the pretense he is full, and almost immediately begins to look for something else to eat, he should note that he was lying to himself. He should return to the last fruit he was eating and deliberately taste it again. He may discover that in fact he doesn't like the taste any more (which is the real reason he stopped eating it). It is rare for anyone to feel "full" on fruits and other native foods — although it is common on hamburgers and french-fries. With original foods, when one has had enough to eat, he doesn't feel "full," he just feels he's had his fill.

If the eater becomes truly satiated during the fruit course, he can simply stop eating, and lunch for him will have been a single course meal. If he's still hungry after finishing one kind of fruit, he can then select another, or go on to the second course. However, once he has started the second course, he should not go back to eating fruit again.

The second course consists of nuts. The same principles apply: each type of food should be smelled in turn (warming them in the hand enhances the smell) and the most attractive one eaten, either until the taste changes or until the eater has truly had his fill. A second type of nut may be selected and eaten after the first one has become unattractive, but the preferred practice restricts consumption to only one kind. (There is no harm in tasting nuts if the smell is too faint to give a clear signal.)

After the nuts come honeys. Again, selection is made by

smell, and the preferred type of honey is eaten until it becomes disagreeable to the palate, or until the eater has had his fill.

Dinner. Dinner may be a one-, two-, three- or four-course meal including the following groups:

1st course — Group 1a: meat or eggs
　　　　　　　or
　　　　　　　Group 1b: seafoods
　　　　　　　or
　　　　　　　Group 4b: germinated seeds and legumes

2nd course — Group 3: vegetables

3rd course — Group 2: fruits

4th course — Group 5: honeys

The method at dinner time is the same as the one used at lunch. However, the evening meal will begin with a selection of foods from *either* Group 1a (animal meats and eggs) *or* 1b (seafoods) *or* 4b (germinated seeds and legumes). These groups are mutually exclusive; they should not be eaten at the same meal. For instance, if one has been eating clams, and the taste goes bad, he should not then switch to lamb or to eggs, or to germinated seeds and legumes.

The reason for not mixing these foods is that each type contains different enzymes, which call for very different types of digestive enzyme production in our bodies. Our systems cannot "do everything at once," so mixing foods from these different groups will usually produce digestive and metabolic problems, sometimes severe.

These first-course foods, although usually classified as "proteins," include much more than what that word refers to. Again, it is impossible to predict the amount a person may eat before his taste actually changes. As a general rule, however, protein consumption under Anopsological conditions amounts to about a third of the quantities generally thought of as "normal." This

would seem to lend some weight to the vegetarian and fructar-
ian arguments that meat is "unnatural" for humans. However,
infants and children, prior to any conditioning, can be seen to
spontaneously select raw meat, fish, and shellfish, and consume
them in relatively large amounts compared to adults. Furthermore, in some cases of severe pathology, and in some cases of
extreme obesity, animal foods may be practically the only kinds
that appeal to the senses, and should be eaten for this very reason.

We might add that *any part* of a fish or animal may smell and
taste attractive, not only muscle fiber. Any organs of fish or land
animals may become attractive to someone when he needs their
nutrients.

This notion may disturb someone more accustomed to looking at food than to actually smelling and tasting it. Should anyone eat foods this way if it upsets him? Certainly not. But anyone
who is willing to explore his reactions, and possibly question a
few taboos, will have pleasures in store beyond anything he
imagined. Once the senses have reawakened, the delight to be
found in a native food the body truly needs can literally border
on ecstasy.

For the squeamish, an easy introduction to eating raw fish
can be had at any Japanese "Sushi" restaurant. Here he will find
delicately cut slices of Yellowtail, Tuna, Salmon, etcetera, served
with rice ("Sushi") or without ("Sashimi") that he can eat in the
company of perfectly normal people, not all of them Japanese,
who enjoy eating well. He can even dip the fish in soy sauce,
and explain to his neighbors that most exceptionally he's cheat-
ing a little on Anopsological practice . . .

The second course at dinner is Group 3, vegetables. These
might include: tomatoes, celery, green peppers, beets, cucumbers, lettuce, broccoli, artichokes. Vegetables can be refrigerated
for storage, but their smells and tastes will be undetectable unless
they are at room temperature. Again, after selecting one kind of
vegetable, it should be eaten until the taste becomes unattractive before going on to another.

The third course is fruits, preferably limited to one or two varieties, selected and eaten in the same manner.

If there is an attraction to it, the meal can be ended with honey.

Some Commercially Available Foods that can be Selected and Eaten by Instinct

Group 1a: Land Animals

Beef	Goose	Rabbit
Chicken	Lamb	Turkey
Duck	Partridge	Veal
Eggs	Pheasant	Etc.
Goat	Pork	

Group 1b: Seafoods

Clams	Redsnapper	Squid
Crab	Sailfish	Tuna
Crayfish	Salmon	Turbot
Fish eggs	Sardines	Trout
Lobster	Sea urchins	Yellowtail
Mussels	Seiche	Etc.
Oysters	Shrimp	

Group 2: Fruits

Apples	Boysenberries	Cherries
Apricots	Cactus pears	Chirimoya
Bananas	Cantaloupe	Coconuts
Blackberries	Carob	Cranberries
Blueberries	Cassia	Currants

Dates
Figs
Gooseberries
Grapefruit
Grapes
Guanabana
Guavas
Kiwi fruit
Kumquats
Lemons
Limes

Litchees
Mangoes
Nectarines
Oranges
Papaya
Passion fruit
Peaches
Pears
Persimmons
Pineapple
Plantanes

Pomegranate
Plums
Prunes
Raisins
Raspberries
Strawberries
Tamarind
Tangerines
Watermelon
Zapote
Etc.

Group 3: Vegetables

Artichokes
Asparagus
Avocados
Beans (fresh)
Beets
Broccoli
Brussels sprouts
Cabbage
Cauliflower
Celeriac
Celery
Chinese cabbage
Corn
Cucumbers
Eggplant

Garlic
Jicama
Kohlrabi
Leeks
Lettuce
Mint
Mushrooms
Okra
Olives
Parsley
Parsnips
Peas, sweet
Peas, chick (fresh)
Peppers
Potatoes

Pumpkin
Radishes
Rhubarb
Rutabaga
Spinach
Squash
String Beans
Sugar cane
Turnips
Watercress
Yams
Zucchini
Etc.

Group 4a: Nuts

Almonds	Coconuts	Pistachios
Brazil nuts	Hazelnuts	Walnuts
Cashews	Peanuts	Etc.
Chestnuts	Pecans	

Group 4b: Seeds & Legumes

Barley	Linseed	Sunflower
Beans (black,	Oats	seeds
red, etc.)	Rye	Etc.
Lentils	Sesame	

Group 5: Honeys & Pollen

Acacia	Eucalyptus	Pine
Clover	Flowers	Etc.

' Edward Howell, *Enzyme Nutrition*, p. 123, Avery Publishing Group, Wayne, N.J., 1985.

Chapter 20

Our Native Foods

Instinctive nutrition functions correctly only with whole foods in their native, original state as found in nature. Our innate, genetically determined alimentary programming did not evolve with respect to separate "nutrients" (i.e., vitamins, minerals, amino acids and other entities identified by laboratory analyses conducted in vitro. Nor can such analyses ever say "everything" about a food (or anything else). Nature will forever remain more complex than the mere convolutions of our brains (and the analytical methods to which they give rise). *The whole is greater than the sum of its parts* is particularly true about food.

Once a food has been denatured, it no longer entirely fits our metabolic needs, even when "fortified" with synthetic or synthesized substances believed to be lacking. When we are dealing with a food in its original state, if too many of the nutrients we need at that moment are missing, we will normally not be attracted to it.

We can know whether an original food is one we need (or in the laboratory vernacular, "contains" what we need) by smelling it. If it smells attractive, that means we need it, and we will want it; otherwise we won't. The general rule is:

THE MORE PLEASURE WE HAVE WITH A FOOD'S SMELL AND TASTE, THE MORE WE NEED IT AND THE MORE IT IS FILLING OUR NEED.

This is not true of denatured foods, that can be artificially made so attractive, and so detrimental for our health, that we need to limit consumption (e.g., butterscotch sundaes).

In the preceding chapter, we recommended that meals proceed one course after another. The intention is that each course should offer a variety of foods among which to "forage," so that only the *most attractive* items (i.e., the most nourishing in terms of the body's needs at that moment) will be eaten. Depending on pocketbook and availability, a course might contain two, five or twenty-five different items belonging to a particular group of foods. The greater the variety, the greater the chance that a person may discover among them, by smell and taste, an item that fills urgent metabolic needs. For a person in fairly good health, there may be no true urgencies, and a limited selection will probably suffice. For someone critically ill, the larger the choice, the better his chances of finding foods that will enable him to recover.

Now we will discuss the food groups separately, along with some of the individual foods within them, and make some suggestions about purchasing, serving and eating them.

Chapter 21

Animal Foods

Group 1a: Land Animals & Eggs

Some current objections to eating meat. It has been argued on philosophical grounds that men should not eat meat because it is immoral to slaughter animals. This issue is closer to theology than nutrition. Each person must choose for himself, and consistently with his beliefs, and we cannot argue with persons eschewing meat for moral reasons.

On other grounds, the argument has been advanced that men were not intended for meat because they lack the incisors and claws of carnivores such as tigers and minks.' Many people have discovered, in fact, that their health improved when they avoided meat. What few of them ever noticed, however, is that their health improved when they were avoiding *cooked* meat. Meat in its native state is a different matter.

It should be noted in passing that men do in fact possess vestigial incisors as well as claws – their fingernails – and it can be reasonably inferred that at some distant point in mankind's evolutionary development, pre-humans and pre-tigers were, if not one and the same, at least close cousins. It should also be noted that some rodents, equipped with both claws and incisors, are predominantly vegetarian rather than carnivorous, and that carnivores may also eat vegetable foods on occasion.

It is regularly seen under Anopsological conditions, that healthy infants and children, as well as adults, are spontaneously attracted to the smells and tastes of meats. But they consume significantly *less* meat than the population at large eating cooked foods. So the inference is warranted that men are *relatively* non-carnivorous, but only relatively so. It would seem, in fact, that many animals may be relatively more omnivorous than is suggested by the either-or categories of classical zoology. Anyone who ever saw chickens feasting on grass, insects, fish heads, carcasses and other chickens' blood (and not only on grains in a trough) would not doubt this.

Vegetarians who wish to practice instinctive nutrition without recourse to meat should do so. One can obtain a great deal of protein from nuts, legumes and other vegetable sources. Vegetable protein is chemically similar to animal protein. But seed foods are not whole-animal foods, and cannot entirely substitute for them.

A critical study of the history of use of foods as curative agents forces one to the conclusion that the virtue of effective foods resides in their possessing all of the nutritional factors nature gave them.[2]

Problems with meat. The most widespread problem with meat comes from what nourished the animals: chemically fertilized corn, or wheat, that is not a native food for cattle; cooked slops that are not native nourishment for hogs; synthetic food supplements; synthetic hormones, and vaccines. These additives produce in animals mismetabolized cellular wastes that cannot be eliminated and which accumulate as fat. The mechanisms of fat accumulation in cattle or pigs reflect those in humans who ingest denatured foods their metabolisms can neither use nor eliminate.

The top grade of U.S. Government Inspected beef comes from animals so overburdened with undischargeable wastes that their flesh is speckled with it. Its price is higher than the leaner grades of beef. It is "the best" — for the cattleman. It may one day be recognized as dangerous for human consumption. Several Western European countries have banned by law, the use of hormones for animals raised for the market. It has been widely understood that residues from fertilizers and pesticides, previously used on fodder sources, wind up in the animals (particularly in the liver and kidneys, but also in the muscle tissue and fat) and subsequently in whoever eats them. Cooking the contaminants only further complicates them chemically; it does not decontaminate them.

Experienced instinctive eaters, whose smell and taste sensitivity is considerably more acute than the average, will generally not eat commercial meat. They will tell you most of it stinks, and carries a bitter, chemical aftertaste.

If meat of any kind smells and tastes unpleasant, it may be because one doesn't need it, or because of unpleasant substances within it. In either case, an unpleasant smell is something any animal in nature will instinctively avoid because it is dangerous, and we too should follow this rule.

One should look for meat that is certified as coming from range-fed animals that received no hormones, fodders, supplements, etc. Fortunately, because of growing demand, there is a growing supply of meat from relatively clean animals. Instinctive eaters will further increase this supply by simply requesting it.

A second danger in uncooked meats comes from parasites. However, among the several thousand people currently practicing instinctual nutrition in France, there have been no reports of parasitic infection. There are two probable reasons for this:

1. Beef that is raised to Anopsological standards is strictly range-fed, with no alimentary additions. As a result, the animals' immune systems function normally; they are resistant to parasitic infection. This also applies to Anopsological hogs, raised exclusively on raw fruits and vegetables that they forage among by instinct. None has ever been found to harbor parasites. Since many French "Instinctos" eat only this kind of meat, they are not exposed to parasites in the first place.

2. The immune system of an instinctive eater also functions normally, and far more energetically, than that of the average mis-nourished person. Most instinctive eaters become immune to infections of almost any kind, parasites included. New instinctive eaters will discover this for themselves in a relatively short time.

Pork poses a special problem because of the worm *Trichinosis*, whose dangers may well lay at the root of the historical injunction against pork in both the Jewish and Moslem religions. Unless one can buy pork that is certified Trichinosis free, or raises pigs himself to Anopsological standards, it is probably wisest to avoid pork altogether. Experienced instinctive eaters do not fear Trichinosis infection as long as they have been maintaining correct instinctive practice. But pork is not advised for beginners, or for part-time instinctive eaters.

Until such a time as meat vendors can certify their products parasite free (which may hopefully happen some day), the beginning instinctive eater might do the following:

a. Avoid meat entirely for two or three weeks, until he feels confident that his immune system has regained enough strength to protect him against possible parasites (even though his biomedical friends might convulse at the idea that someone could evaluate his own immunological state better than they can)

or

b. continue to cook it, but eat it very rare. If he was doing this already, he may *not* have been killing worm larvae, but he probably didn't realize it and so didn't fear them. As explained above, he should fear them even less if he is eating all his other food by instinct.

If one is afraid of eating "undercooked" meat, or finds it distasteful, he can still make good use of his instinct for food by eating as many other foods as possible according to Anopsological principles. He will be unable to judge correctly whether his body needs meat at all, or how much to eat (unless he eats enough to make him "full," which would probably be excessive and toxic).

He will have to judge how much he can easily digest, and which will not leave him feeling unwell.

How to eat meat. A meat course might consist, for instance, of an assortment of beef steak, beef liver, lamb chop, lamb kidney, chicken thigh, turkey breast and chicken eggs. They can be laid out separately on a large platter or on small plates. A few thin slices may be prepared separately for smelling and tasting, laid out like cold-cuts. Linen and silverware are by no means taboo.

The meat course includes a number of different items so that we can compare their *relative attractiveness* in order to eat only the one we need most. The first step, then, is to sniff each item closely in turn before tasting any of them. The second step will be to taste the food that smelled best, and the third will be to eat it, a bite at a time, until the taste veers from good to bad. At that point the meat course is finished and after a few minute's rest, the next one can begin.

If a food smelled good, but did not taste good, it should not be eaten, and the smell-testing can resume with the remaining items. If none of the items smell good, or none taste good, it means there was nothing among them that the body needed. There is no reason to be concerned when this happens, even if it happens repeatedly for days or even weeks on end; the organism knows what it needs at a given moment, and it may not even be listed in the familiar "Minimum Daily Requirement" tables.

At the outset, if two or more items seem to smell equally good, they should be tested again by smell, one after the other, until one or another stands out clearly as the most attractive. This may seem tedious at first, but it is easy to do, and after a few meals it becomes automatic.

A few words are in order regarding raw meat in particular (but that apply to fish as well) because so many people seem to have a preconceived aversion to eating it.

Anyone may occasionally be more upset by his representation of events to come, than by the events themselves when they finally occur. This is particularly true for someone who has long been eating denatured foods that ennervate the nervous system and produce anxiety. His problem will be not so much how to deal with raw foods, as how to deal with the *idea* of raw foods.

If one gives his imagination free reign, and fantasizes about dangling tendons, torn cartilage, and dripping blood, he may very well want to throw up. The truth of the matter is that almost every modern-day instinctive eater, at some early point, had to face revulsive feelings, *not* with respect to any products of nature, but to the products of his imagination. However, *imagined* horrors can often be more painful than even the cruelest realities.

We are oriented in our culture to *looking* at foods. This is why food coloring is used, why special filtered lights are set up to illuminate meat displays, why produce is polished and waxed. These marketing techniques both exploit and reinforce our visual bias, but they lead us astray. Visual cues, for humans and most other mammals, serve essentially to locate potential food, not to determine whether it is edible. Only smell and taste can serve that function.

If we can reduce, even slightly, our obsession with the visual aspects of food, we will soon stop discovering fantasy ogres beyond the rims of our frying pans.

A world of unbelievable pleasure awaits those who will dare close their eyes momentarily and open their noses and mouths. There is an easy way to start: by using a blindfold (it's too tempting to peek just closing one's eyes). Sleep-masks are cheap and easily found, and while one person wears one, the other can present under his nose, one by one, morsels of food to be smelled. When the masked person has found the one he prefers, he can remove the blindfold and eat it himself, or the other can cut and feed it to him bite by bite, until he reports that the taste has changed.

Kids love to do it, and adults will too, once they discover how rewarding it can be.

Meat taste. Meat that smells attractive may sometimes not taste good. When the body needs it, the taste is sweet and rich, becoming bitter or going flat when one has had his fill. Unless a piece of meat tastes delicious (not just vaguely pleasant or acceptable) it should not be eaten. This applies to the meat and organs of all land animals including fowl.

Storage. Anopsologically raised meat does not spoil as fast as contaminated meat. When good meat can be found, one may wish to buy an extra supply to keep on hand. It can be kept refrigerated with separate unwrapped pieces hung from wire hooks (paper clips will work) with space between them for air circulation. The surface will dry out somewhat, but remain edible.

With time, meat will begin to smell stronger. Persons who regularly eat by instinct will usually find the smell of aged meat *more* attractive than the relatively bland odor of fresh meat. Naturally, what one person might call a stench, for another might be a delight.

Meat can also be preserved by drying it. Thin slices can be laid on a coarse wire mesh and dried at room temperature in a draft (a fan can be used). The jerky made this way will continue to produce an alliesthetic response when one has eaten all he needs.

Rinsing meat. Rinsing meat under running water will destroy much of its smell and taste. This question is discussed later in this chapter.

Eggs

Problems with eggs. The most frequently heard objection to eggs is that they contain cholesterol and are dangerous for the heart and arteries, particularly in persons who already have high cholesterol levels. Cholesterol accumulations result, however, from *cooked* fats; they *decrease* when *raw* fats and egg yolks are eaten.

> . . . *when fats, either animal or vegetable, are eaten along with their associated enzymes, no harmful effect on the arteries or heart results. All fatty foods contain lipase in their natural state. Cooking or processing removes it.*[3]

These remarks about chicken eggs apply to eggs from any fowl.

165

Commercial eggs from malnourished chickens should be avoided if possible. One should seek "organic" eggs from free-roaming chickens that were not nourished on chemically fertilized wheat and corn. A choice between fertilized or unfertilized eggs should be based on which ones taste better.

Eggs may be kept under refrigeration, but should be eaten at room temperature; they can be "ultra-soft-boiled" to take off the chill without cooking them.

Egg taste. Eggs can rarely be tested by odor except in a hen-house. The white and the yolk should be *tasted separately* with a spoon. Generally, the yolk will taste attractive more frequently than the white. Neither should be eaten unless they are patently delicious. When the yolk changes taste, it will become bland or sour. The white will taste sweet when the body needs it, becoming neutral when the need has been filled.

Group 1b: Seafoods

Problems with seafoods. The major problem with seafoods is water pollution. There is little an individual can do about it except avoid eating seafood when toxicity warnings are issued. Commercially grown fresh-water fish should be avoided, since they are raised on chemical fodders.

How to eat fish. Lessons in the art of preparing and eating raw fish can be had by watching the preparers at a Japanese "Sushi" bar. But the carvers usually prepare only filets and throw the rest of the fish away. Any part of a fish, clam, lobster, or crab, can taste delicious when the body needs it. Beginners will probably restrict themselves to flesh for a while, but when they are ready for it they should try smelling and tasting the heads, bones, and livers.

Seafoods should be purchased fresh, i.e., not previously frozen. Larger fish may be rinsed before being cut open, but *once they are open they should not be rinsed.* The reason is that running water carries away smell and taste . . . and nutrients. Filets or other pieces of fish should be *wiped* clean with a cloth or paper towel if desired. Smaller fish, such as sardines, should not be rinsed at all – it will thoroughly destroy their smell, and the taste will be ruined. After the heads and entrails are removed they should simply be wiped clean and laid out on a plate.

The following comments on nutrient loss in washed rice apply to any food, and are particularly applicable to fish:

> *Nutrient loss during food preparation may occur not only as a result of peeling or trimming foods, but through such seemingly harmless procedures as cleansing with a water rinse . . . The fact that as much as one-fourth of a nutrient (available iron) may be lost is quite alarming when one considers how diligently the housewife washes many foods.*[4]

An accompanying table showed a loss of riboflavin of 16.9%, calcium 10%, niacin 9.1%, phosphorous 4.7%.

The fluids contained in shellfish are highly nutritious, and should not be washed down the drain. The juices in oysters and clams should be consumed along with the flesh. Lemon juice should not be used since it prevents proper evaluation of the food's taste.

Seafood taste. The taste-change phenomenon varies greatly between one seafood and another, and may involve texture as well as taste. Tuna, for example, may become "gluey" in the mouth. Clams, oysters and other shellfish may become bitter, acrid, or the eater may suddenly become thirsty, which means that he has reached a saturation point for salt and should stop. Scallops may become over-sweet, while crab may change from sweet to acrid. The taste-change in most seafoods occurs rapidly and is clear-cut, probably because animal life from the sea is truly in its native state, unmodified by selective breeding.

Preserving seafoods. Most seafoods can be kept fresh for a few days under refrigeration, protecting them from the air (shellfish do not require wrapping). Fish filets can be dried, however, in the same way as meat, on a coarse mesh at room temperature in a draft. Although they may smell strongly for a while, the smell will subside once they are dry. Fish dried this way will produce an alliesthetic response like fresh fish.

[1] Herbert Shelton, *The Science and Fine Art of Food and Nutrition*, The Natural Hygiene Press, Oldsmar, 1984.

[2] Edward Howell, *Enzyme Nutrition*, op. cit. p. 101.

[3] Edward Howell, *Enzyme Nutrition*, op. cit. p. 148.

[4] Harris and Loesecke, *Nutritional Evaluation of Food Processing*, John Wiley & Sons, New York, 1960.

Chapter 22

Group 2: Fruit

Problems with fruit. Once again, the major problem with fruit concerns contaminants: chemical fertilizers, insecticides and preservatives. Irradiation is also a problem.

Since Anopsological practice rapidly increases smell and taste sensitivity, most people should soon have little difficulty knowing whether the fruits on their table are contaminated or not: the ones raised on chemical fertilizers carry the taste.

Irradiated fruit will not ripen, and its smell and taste will be altered and weakened. If fruit at room temperature for a week or more does not noticeably mature, it should be returned to the store and the storekeeper challenged to eat it himself.

Most fruit in American supermarkets has had its skin sprayed, waxed, or deodorized. The shopper will usually have to scratch the skin with a fingernail in order to smell it, to decide whether to buy it. Once this practice becomes current, store managers may begin to put out samples for shoppers to test.

Eventually this might force growers to ship fruit more worthy of the name.

> *A detailed examination revealed . . . that in a number of instances the variety of a food plant produced in Mexico or Central America was higher in nutritional value than the same food grown in the United States . . . . In his desire to produce lovelier apples, sweeter oranges, blander vegetables, ship-resistant foods, he has often produced varieties which are less nutritious per pound.*

Fruits in season. The argument has been advanced that only locally grown fruits should be eaten, and only in season, because this is the natural way of man's harmony with his environment. Let us assume it is true. If it is, then bananas are a perfectly harmonious food in Milwaukee in January, when the inhabitants are spending most of their time inside buildings or clothes that maintain their skins at the temperature of Devil's Island at daybreak. Man-made environments are just as real as "real" ones, and call for harmony too.

Storage. In general, tropical fruits may be damaged by refrigeration, and should be kept at room temperature, close to their native ambient temperature. Many of them, such as bananas, peaches, grapes, and figs, can be dried in the same way as meat or fish: on wire mesh in a draft, in the shade. Drying them in hot air or in the sun will cook them, destroy their taste-change potential and make them toxic to a degree.

Eating fruit. Because commercially grown fruit is artificially bred to taste *better* than its wild cousins in nature, it takes longer for its taste to turn bad, so we may eat more than we need unless we compensate for this factor. The way to do this is to *stop eating fruit when the taste becomes neutral,* before it becomes sharply distasteful. This should be taken as a general rule with fruit in an everyday (non-therapeutic) context. The problem is less critical than with vegetables, and is therefore examined in greater detail in the section, "Problems with vegetables."

The following remarks do not apply to fruits that have been irradiated:

Apples. Taste fades and texture becomes mushy. Scratch the skin of waxed apples to obtain a smell. Overripe apples can be delicious when a person needs them and should be tested by smell.

Bananas. Bananas that are speckled were shipped in a gas environment to artificially ripen them and should be avoided if possible. Naturally ripened bananas carry black streaks and blotches, but few speckles. Both green and overripe bananas may sometimes be more attractive than bananas that seem ideally ripe, and should be tested by smell, then by taste. At the turning point, taste disappears and texture becomes mushy.

Berries. Many hard-skinned berries do not carry a strong smell and should be tested by taste; the meat can be spit out if it is unappealing. Berries should be wiped clean of pesticides rather than rinsed. Most berries will taste acid when the body doesn't need them, but the senses will be misled if sugar is added. Adding sugar makes it possible to avoid having left-over berries that might be wasted. But it also makes it possible to develop "allergic" reactions so a few wasted berries is preferable. Preferably, eat only one kind of berry at a meal.

Cactus Pears. Watch out for the little spines in the skin — they should be removed entirely before eating. This fruit is very tasty when needed, turning bland when the stop-point is reached.

Cantaloupe. See Melons.

Carob. Natural Carob batons can be cut open and chewed if the taste is good. Natural Carob might not be as appealing as someone accustomed to Carob-coated raisins might expect. Also, this fruit often has a constipating effect, and should be tested regularly by anyone suffering from loose bowels.

Cassia (Sena). This naturally occurring gourd grows wild from tropical Mexico south. It looks like a hand-rolled cigar about two feet long. The gourd contains compartments with seeds in them, separated by small disks coated with a black licorice-like substance that can smell delicious or rotten depending on need. The disks are licked until the taste begins to bite the tongue and throat.

This fruit was used as a natural laxative in Europe at the beginning of the century. It contributes greatly to metabolic detoxination, and should be tested regularly, if possible *outside of mealtimes,* just before going to bed or upon getting up. It may provoke diarrhea at first that later becomes infrequent.

Cassia is such an effective "cleanser" that it should be regularly used by anyone who is making a serious effort to recover his health through instinctive nutrition. It is mandatory for any systematic Anopsotherapy program.

Cherries. Difficult to smell; should be tested by taste. Become bland/acid when no longer needed.

Chirimoya. This semi-tropical fruit is the size of a small musk melon with flesh the texture of cotton. Superb when the body needs it, becoming "stinky" when it doesn't. May produce strong detoxination reactions. Rarely available in the U.S.

Citrus Fruits. Cut fruit along the "equator," then quarter the hemispheres. Let the lips come in contact with the skin, and eat everything inside, including the pith (but not the seeds). This applies to all citrus fruits.

Dates. Fresh dates become sour when no longer needed. Commercially dried dates are generally dried at high temperature and should be avoided since they can easily be eaten to excess, producing "allergic" reactions and malaise. Buy dried dates only if the seller can certify that they were air-dried, and only if they produce a sweet-to-sour taste change.

Figs. When no longer needed, fresh figs will turn "uncomfortable" in the mouth. The remarks about dried dates also apply to dried figs.

Grapefruit. All varieties can be eaten, but the white-flesh, seed-bearing kind produce the strongest alliesthetic reaction. See Citrus Fruits.

Grapes. All varieties produce an alliesthetic response, although it is milder in seedless grapes. They should be tested by tasting since they carry little smell. The seeds may be eaten or not according to individual preference. Grapes become acid and/or bitter when not needed.

Guava. Sweet when needed, otherwise acid. Can be cut in half and eaten with a teaspoon, seeds included.

Kiwi. This fruit is very sweet when needed, becoming acrid and pungent when enough has been eaten. Kiwis are best eaten cut lengthwise into quarters, the flesh cut or spooned away from the skin, otherwise the skin will burn the lips.

Kumquats. Can be chewed up and eaten whole. Become unpleasantly bitter when not needed.

Lemons, Limes. Delicious eaten whole like grapefruit when needed, becoming acid. See Citrus Fruits.

Litchees. Sometimes called the "Cherries of Asia." The husk is peeled away, the flesh torn from the single central seed. Highly aromatic, very sweet changing to sour.

Mangoes. Mangoes cultivated by artificial selection have relatively smooth flesh; wild mangoes as a rule are smaller and stringy, with stronger smell and taste. Mangoes should be tested by smell where the stalk meets the fruit. Underripe mangoes are acid with a turpentine-like flavor. Quarter the skin and pull it in sections away from the flesh (but don't waste the flesh that adheres to it). The remainder can be cut, chewed, or sucked, in any way that works. The alliesthetic response is clear, even with cultivated varieties.

Melons. Watch out for fertilizer after-taste. Most melons, including watermelons, have a sweet-to-sour taste change. Melons should be eaten ripe and at room temperature, cut in any way that is convenient.

Nectarines. Although Nectarines were first produced by hybridization between peaches and plums, they produce a clear-cut taste change to acid. Can be peeled if pesticides are feared. Best eaten ripe.

Oranges. Many varieties exist, and either "juice" oranges or "eating" oranges may taste best. Test by smelling scratched-out spot on skin. See Citrus Fruits.

Papaya. The small varieties can be cut in half lengthwise and eaten with a spoon, with or without the seeds. Test by smell, which may be strongly revulsive when body doesn't need it. Taste changes from delicious to bland.

Passion Fruit. Numerous varieties exist, lemon-sized dark green, orange-sized light yellow, and so on. Test by cutting open and smelling. Fabulously delicious when needed, unbearably acid when the stop-point is reached.

Peaches. All varieties become bland/sour when need has been filled. Test by smell. Organically grown peaches are preferable, with commercial peaches watch out for chemical after-taste.

Pears. All varieties should be tested by smell. Taste-change is mild; pears become "uninteresting."

Persimmons. The well-known puckering effect of Persimmons is the alliesthetic reaction. After a person's organism has become cleansed of some of its denatured-food toxins, as many as five or ten persimmons, even unripe, might be consumed before the taste changes. Should be cut open and tested by smell and taste.

Pineapple. Many varieties abound, from different sources. Avoid fruit that carries a fertilizer after-taste. Generally, the smaller in size, the better the taste, but some exceptions occur. Eat pineapple ripe. The top can be twisted off, and the exposed fruit tested by smell. Pineapples are best cut in half *lengthwise,* the hemispheres then cut into wedges. Some of the core fiber can be cut off along the top of each wedge (it is bitter and would be spit out anyway), then a series of small perpendicular cuts can be made an inch apart along the wedge to produce convenient bite-size sections. Pineapples produce a ferocious taste-change reaction, become acid/biting.

Plantane. This reddish variety of banana is usually cooked, but tastes excellent raw to someone who needs it. Should be tested by taste; becomes flat-tasting and starchy when need is filled.

Pomegranate. Can be halved or quartered and the seeds picked out in batches with the teeth. Puckers the mouth when the taste-change is reached; at this point, beware the temptation to crush and suck seeds for their juice only, which will still taste good. The excess will produce toxic reactions.

Plums. All varieties produce a fairly good alliesthetic response, usually an acid increase or loss of flavor. Wipe clean or peel if the skin tastes bad.

Prunes are dried plums, and are universally heat-dried in commerce and produce no taste-change. To be avoided unless one makes his own. Plums are not needed to facilitate intestinal passage of foods when a person is eating instinctively. Natural prunes will not produce diarrhea (i.e., act like "natural laxatives") because they will not be eaten to excess.

Raisins are dried grapes, and are also heat-dried in commerce. Same comments as prunes.

Tamarind. Small flat shell pulls apart to reveal reddish brown, fudge-like flesh, with strong pungent odor becoming unbearably acid when no longer needed. Traditionally used as a laxative, but cannot be eaten to diarrhea-producing excess in its natural state.

Watermelon. See Melons.

Zapote. Black flesh of *"Zapote Negro"* can be luscious, becoming bland/acid when enough has been eaten. White variety becomes biting. Rarely available in the U.S.

' Harris and Loesecke, op. cit.

Chapter 23

Group 3:
Vegetables

Problems with vegetables

Here again a major problem with vegetables is pollution. Chemical fertilizers, insecticides, and preservative sprays all find their way ultimately into the body of the consumer. Nothing much need be added to our previous discussions of this problem. We can only wipe, cut, scrape, and rinse away the contaminants as best we can. Thoroughly soaking and washing vegetables should be avoided since it removes many valuable nutrients and kills taste and smell.

Another major problem arises as a result of artificial selection. In their efforts to increase profits, growers have for many years been developing special strains of produce designed to stand up better during shipment, resist infection, and be visually more attractive. They also sought to enhance a bland taste in the varieties that are normally eaten raw (e.g., cucumbers, tomatoes). These are the ones that sell best because weak vegetables produce weak alliesthetic reactions, and consumers therefore eat more of them.

Vegetables destined for cooking (or canning, or freezing), on the other hand, are artificially selected for their attractiveness *after* denaturation. The result is that most *raw* vegetables on the market are *less* attractive than they would be if they had never been tampered with. They are relatively so unattractive, in fact, that unless we know how to compensate for it, we may end up eating so few that we deprive ourselves of nutrients that only vegetables can provide. Fancy dressings are not the answer. If we can, we need to account for the calculated imbalance of vegetables, and it is easy to do so once we understand how our taste-change works in relation to them.

The following diagram shows typical taste-change patterns for three vegetables: leeks, tomatoes and yams.

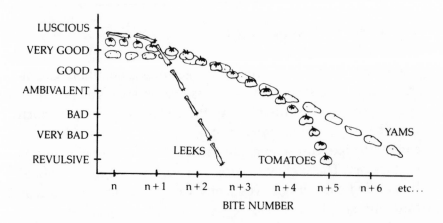

Leeks:

Tomatoes:

Yams:

A person's innate biochemical programming both imparts a good taste to a native food when it is needed, and causes it to turn bad when need has been filled. "Good" and "Bad" are not absolutes, however. The vertical axis in this drawing shows a continuum from "delicious" to "revulsive," but these feelings are relative to each other, not to some hypothetical absolute standard. They necessarily reflect different intensities of sensation for different foods, and for different individuals at different times.

The horizontal axis represents the amount of food eaten in terms of number of "bites." We cannot know in advance whether a change in taste will occur with the third bite (or "mouthful," or "morsel") or the twenty-third or the sixtieth, so "n" represents an unknown variable. It enables us simply to represent a taste-change without specifying how much might be eaten before it occurs.

Ideally, a person would stop eating a food as its changing taste passed through the mid-point, and before it became sharply revulsive. This should theoretically insure a perfect match between need and fulfillment. In practice, however, vestigial organic maladjustments will long persist to distort the equation on the "demand" side, while the "supply" side is thrown off by artificial selection.

It was mentioned earlier that fruits are raised to be *more* attractive than they would be in nature, so the eater should stop when their taste becomes "mildly good," *before* it goes flat or "bad." But vegetables are bred to make them unnaturally *less* attractive when raw, so the opposite applies. In other words, the eater should ideally eat vegetables, not until the "neutral" point is reached, but *until the taste has become clearly unpleasant.*

Storage

Vegetables keep best if refrigerated, but wrapping them in plastic is not the best way to store them. Unless they can "breathe" they will begin to rot, and they will wither unless they are kept moist. Vegetables, particularly the leafy ones, are best kept wrapped in damp dish-cloths.

Eating Vegetables

As with other foods, alliesthetic reactions vary greatly between one type of vegetable and another. Vegetables should be eaten at room temperature. Some vegetables are best eaten in a particular way. Vegetables can best be tested by smell by scratching or making a cut in the skin.

The following remarks do not apply to vegetables that have been irradiated:

Artichokes. Artichokes must be tested by taste. Only the base of the leaves and the heart are eaten. Cut lengthwise (in the direction stalk to pointed tip) into quarters. Remove the fuzz from the heart. Eat the bases of the leaves, working toward the heart. Fabulously delicious when the body needs it, but former consumers of cooked artichokes may not find raw ones attractive for some time. Sharp rapid taste change from delicious to piquant or biting.

Asparagus. Should be tested by taste. The stem is much tastier than the flower. Taste slowly becomes sour.

Avocado. Many varieties available. Can be tested by smell; if no odor detected then it will probably not taste good. Cut in half and eat with a spoon. Taste becomes slowly uninteresting, unpleasant.

Beans. Fresh beans from the pod can be eaten like peas, but are generally not a favorite vegetable. Taste becomes sour, unpleasant. Should be tested by smell and taste.

Broccoli. Usually necessary to test by taste. The flowers are practically tasteless; the food is the stalks. When enough has been eaten, broccoli becomes biting.

Brussels Sprouts. Necessary to test by taste. Sweet when needed, becoming very sour.

Cabbage. Red or Green cabbage, test by smell and taste. The base of the leaf is tastiest. Delicious when needed, becoming biting.

Cauliflower. Same comments as Broccoli.

Celeriac. Scratch or cut and test by smell. Becomes sharp when no longer needed.

Celery. Scratch skin and test by smell. Strong taste change: becomes quickly intolerable.

Chinese Cabbage. Test by smell and taste. When not needed becomes bitter and "tastes like cardboard."

Corn. All varieties of sweet corn are edible; must be tested by taste. Delicacy of taste will surprise former cooked-corn lovers. Perfectly delicious when body needs it, becoming slowly uninteresting then inedible when enough has been eaten.

Cucumbers. Test by smell. Need not be peeled. Become acrid when no longer needed.

Eggplant. Test by taste. Most people never find raw eggplant attractive, but some swear by it. Tastes like plaster when not needed.

Garlic. Smell only. If the smell is *strongly attractive,* enjoy the smell until it subsides or turns bad, but do not taste. It is providing valuable aromatic nutrition. If the smell is *mildly* attractive, put garlic to tongue. Eat it *if the taste is not biting,* and spit it out immediately when the taste does become biting. This means the body doesn't need it.

Jicama. Test by taste. Changes from mild sweet taste to pungent "earth-like" flavor.

Kohlrabi. Test by smell and taste. Pleasant taste becomes unpleasantly strong, fairly fast transition.

Leeks. The same comments as garlic: smell only if odor is strong. Leek taste-change is phenomenally rapid; spit out as soon as it occurs.

Lettuce. Test by smell and taste. Becomes uninteresting, slightly sour.

Mint. Crush in fingers and enjoy smell for awhile before tasting. Becomes bitter when not needed.

Mushrooms. Mushrooms are technically not vegetable plants, but are best eaten as part of a vegetable course. TEST BY SMELL. Do not taste if no smell or unattractive smell. Some people peel mushrooms, most don't bother. Taste changes to neutral or variably distasteful depending on variety. Stop eating as soon as this occurs.

Okra. Same comments as eggplant.

Parsley. Crush in fingers and test by smell. If attractive, taste. Becomes bitter when no longer needed.

Parsnips. Test by smell and taste. Fairly fast taste-change to "unbearably strong."

Peas, sweet. Test by smell and taste. Become bland/sour when no longer needed.

Peas, chick. Test by smell and taste. Become sour, starchy.

Peppers. Test by smell. Red, Green and Yellow Bell Peppers are aromatic and very different from one another. They become bitter when not needed. Hot peppers become hot when the taste changes.

Potatoes. Test by smell and taste. Most conveniently eaten in thin slices. Persons not overloaded from a long history of cooked potatoes will find them very attractive on occasion, reverting to a "raw potato" taste when not needed.

Pumpkin. Test by smell and taste. Sweet, almost like melon, when needed, otherwise reverts to sour/starchy.

Radishes. Test by smell. If taste is mildly but pleasantly biting, keep going; abandon when bite becomes strong.

Rhubarb. Test by smell and taste. Aromatic sweetness becoming piquant.

Rutabaga. Test by smell and taste. Becomes sour/biting when not needed.

Spinach. Test by taste. Will become sour and puckering when not needed.

Squash. Same comments as eggplant.

String Beans. Test by taste. Become unpleasantly "grassy" when unneeded.

Sugar Cane. Not technically a vegetable, not a fruit either. Cut away outer husk, test by smell. Chew on cane but spit out excess fiber. Becomes distastefully sweet when not needed.

Turnips. Test by smell. Become sour and biting when not needed.

Watercress. Same comments as parsley.

Yams. Test by smell. Best eaten like potatoes. Delicious for people who need them, otherwise unpleasantly bland.

Zucchini. Same comments as eggplant.

Chapter 24

Nuts & Honeys

Group 4a: Nuts

Problems with nuts. The major problem with nuts is that until they have germinated they contain enzyme inhibitors that make them difficult to evaluate and digest. Even so, they contain many valuable nutrient trace elements, and should be tested regularly for appeal.

A second problem is the way nuts are treated in commerce. For instance, walnuts from the tree are dark brown with uneven coloration and taste strong and fruity. By the time they reach the store, in most cases, they have been bleached, giving them a "clean" anemic hue and a deadened, if not patently bitter, taste. Theoretically, such nuts are better than no nuts at all, but instinctive eaters will not enjoy them. They might do well to badger their suppliers to make *natural* "natural" nuts available – which applies to peanuts, almonds, and other nuts as well.

Another aspect of this problem is what happens to *shelled* raw nuts, a favorite in "Natural" food stores. Once the shells are removed, the oils in the nuts become oxydized and smell rancid. Plastic bags will not prevent it. Here again, the instinctive eater will need to seek out sources of authentic nuts in their original shells, the ones they were born in. What the merchant loses selling "convenience" packages he can make up by selling nutcrackers.

Until germinated nuts are available on the market, consumers will have to germinate their own or make do with nuts that are relatively difficult to digest. Peanuts can be germinated by covering them with a damp cloth in a warm place (see comments below on germinating seeds). Other nuts are technically difficult to germinate readily since they require controlled humidity and temperature conditions not easily reproduced in the home.

How to test nuts. Take a handful of nuts in the palms of your hands, put them close to your mouth and blow on them a few times. That will warm and moisten them and give them an odor. If the smell is not attractive, the taste will not be attractive.

Alternatively, nuts can be soaked for a few hours, or stored in a damp cloth for a day or two. This makes them more aromatic and sometimes tastier.

A detailed discussion of different varieties of nuts is not necessary because of the relative similarity between them. The kinds most often available in a *natural* "natural" state are:

ALMONDS (Hard- and soft-shelled varieties)

BRAZIL NUTS

CHESTNUTS (Available in the autumn, must be eaten fresh)

HAZELNUTS

PEANUTS

PECANS

PISTACHIOS

WALNUTS - BLACK WALNUTS

A Special Case: Coconuts

Coconuts are one of the few foods that have not been denatured by artificial selection and are not denatured in commerce. For this alone they should be highly prized. Coconut milk is abundant in the green fruit — less so in the ripe ones shipped to market — and changes from sweet to bland/sour when no longer needed. In the immature fruit, the meat is soft and can be eaten with a spoon, becoming sour when the taste changes. Meat from a mature coconut can be eaten like the meat of any other nut, becoming sour and "mushy" when the taste changes.

Once opened, coconut meat becomes rancid within hours, but can be wrapped in plastic to delay this for a day or two.

Coconuts can be tested at the market by pulling aside the straw-like hair that often remains over the three "eyes," and smelling the husk. One of the three eyes is soft, and can easily be pierced with an ice-pick or screwdriver and a straw inserted. Once the milk has been drunk, the coconut can be split by hitting it with a hammer or frying pan — in memory of the sizzling sounds of days gone by . . .

Group 4b: Seeds & Legumes

Problems with seeds & legumes. For the most part, these foods were not exposed to the ravages of insecticides but may have been subject to preservatives. They can be tested by blowing on a handful and smelling. Reject them if there are unnatural odors (from the seeds, not the hands — wash hands and *rinse thoroughly* before handling seeds).

Cereals. Wheat is not used in instinctive nutrition because it does not produce a taste change to signal when enough has been eaten. Any other cereal grains can be used *if they are sprouted*. The grains should be spread on a wet cloth and covered with another one, and kept damp and warm until the sprouts appear. At that point they can be tested by smell, and eaten like any other native food until the taste changes.

The cereals most commonly used are OATS, BARLEY and RYE. The adventurous may wish to try sprouting RICE and MILLET as well.

Seeds. The seeds most commonly eaten by instinctive eaters are SUNFLOWER SEEDS and LINSEED. Theoretically they should be sprouted, but this is difficult to do. Therefore they are usually tested and eaten dry, although they can also be soaked. They are generally attractive in small amounts, and this is fortunate because unless they are sprouted, they are difficult to digest.

Legumes. The following can easily be sprouted using the method discussed above:

Beans (dried, all kinds)

Chick Peas

Lentils

Once the sprouts are a quarter to half an inch long they are ready for eating.

Alternatively, legumes can be soaked in water until they are swollen, then eaten like nuts. They are difficult to digest, but some people sometimes enjoy a few this way.

Group 5: Honey & Pollen

Problems with honey. The major problem with honey is fraud. "Natural" honey is the only kind there is, so that even when it has been processed industrially, it is still labelled "natural." However, honey is extremely sensitive to heat, and a temperature only a few degrees higher than the one prevailing inside the hive will denature it enough to prevent a taste change.

Honey that is still in the comb is truly "natural" in the Anopsological sense. It is also natural if it was extracted from the comb by centrifuging (i.e., by artificial gravity), then spooned directly into jars and stored at ambient temperature. The condition is that the honey in the jar came *from a single hive.* Mixed honey from different hives will not produce a correct alliesthetic reaction.

Industrial honey is inevitably a mixture of honeys, which for the most part were extracted from the comb by melting them. At the factory, the honey will again be heated to liquify it for convenience in mixing, and filling jars or cans. Once treated this way, honey remains relatively fluid; it loses the heavy consistency it would have in its native state. It also loses the ability to produce a proper alliesthetic response: it can be eaten until it makes the eater nauseous, whereas original honey produces a taste change and/or burning sensations that prevent excessive ingestion.

Fraud is also practiced by bee-keepers who give refined sugar to their bees after removing so much honey that the hive would starve to death otherwise. Some ingenious bee-keepers have also been known to feed the bees fruit jams to produce exotic flavors that do not exist in nature. With a little experience, the instinctive eater can detect denatured honey almost at once when tasting them.

Honey is generally named for some particular type of vegetation, or in a particular environment in which bees feed. Some examples are:

acacia honey, eucalyptus honey, clover honey, mixed flowers honey, mountain honey, prairie honey, pine forest honey, sagebrush honey, chestnut honey, apple orchard honey, cherry orchard honey, etc.

An assortment of honey should be kept, and tested by smell. Their attractiveness will vary greatly from day to day, and only the best-smelling one should be tasted. It can be eaten as the last course at any meal, and can also be eaten without ill effect as a snack, whenever desired. It is not a good idea to eat two or three different honeys in quick succession.

Any bottled honey whose label does not state unequivocally that it is unmixed, and unheated above hive temperature, should be avoided. Bottled honey with a piece of honeycomb floating in it is suspect, particularly if the label gives no explanation.

The same remarks apply to pollen. Truly natural pollen is delicious for a number of mouthfuls, and then changes taste. If the label does not state categorically that it has never been denatured in any way, it should be left on the shelf.

Chapter 25

What to Expect

It will amaze many people to discover how profoundly nutrition affects them. Although they may have tried various "diets" in the past, no diet will have had the profound effects that original foods produce, when consumed in kind and amount determined by the organism's own biochemistry. It might be helpful to know what to expect.

Instinctual eating is *not* the same thing as eating *raw foods*. Salads are raw, but because they are mixtures, the senses cannot tell which of the ingredients are needed and which are not. Munching on apples "when you feel like it," or downing raw steaks is not the way to use instinct. If a person wants results he should learn to do it correctly.

The key to feeding oneself correctly is: *pleasure*. Many people will have to learn to accept it without guilt. With denatured foods, pleasure often leads to trouble. We may enjoy strawberries & cream, chocolates, buttered popcorn & soft drinks, and almost inevitably pay a price: nausea, indigestion, a "hung over" feeling, hives and so on. As a consequence, in our "normal" nutritional universe, we come to believe that what is pleasurable "isn't good for us," and that for something to be "good for us," it must *not* be pleasurable.

With original foods, just the opposite is true. In nature, what an animal wants is one and the same as what it needs. This applies to humans also. If someone does not enjoy a food, he will not want it, and he shouldn't because *if he doesn't enjoy it he doesn't need it.*

For the first few days, most people do not enjoy original food as much as food that is cooked and seasoned. Their senses of smell and taste are still dull. They are desensitized in part by mis-metabolites still in the body, which came from the processed foods eaten previously. Until this unnatural material is cleaned out, the senses remain denatured too. They will progressively become much more acute, and along with them, eyesight, intuition, and hearing. Thinking should become clearer too. But all this will not happen overnight, and the newcomer will need to be patient and persevere. Once he "gets the hang" of instinctual nutrition, it becomes second nature. After all, it was already with us when we were born, even though it was thwarted.

Within a short time, one will notice that the taste of a food varies with practically every bite. It will feel *alive* — and it is, because natural processes are still at work in original foods. Cooking food or irradiating it stops these processes; they kill food. After a time most people discover that the cooked, seasoned foods they enjoyed previously now taste *dead.* Within two or three weeks, if a person is making no dietary transgressions, he will probably be enjoying original foods more than he enjoyed denatured ones.

If, from the beginning, a person makes no exceptions to eating native foods *exclusively* selected by smell and taste (not by "thinking"), it will become fairly easy for him to eat regularly this way with ever-increasing pleasure. Once the senses have opened up, one may experience extraordinary pleasure with food the body needs. However, dietary transgressions ("oh, just a single candy bar won't hurt anything,") will have the effect of desensitizing the palate. When the next meal is less satisfying, temptation is increased to have another snack on the side, which in turn will cause less enjoyment at the next meal, and so on in a vicious circle. Once a person starts making dietary exceptions, he may quickly find himself back where he started.

From the very first day, *detoxination phenomena* will appear. Let us explain this.

Incorrectly processed molecules from denatured foods – mismetabolites – accumulate in the body as a result of denatured food that could not be used and eliminated correctly. These are molecules that were stripped of some of their radicals, or atoms, and became "stuck" in the metabolism, like a car in a ditch.

Proper food will start things moving again. The body will begin to eliminate the toxic "junk," and more often than not its origins will be clear from the smell. In the past, detoxination programs of this type were probably "treated" with drugs to stop them. If there had not been an enormous amount of "junk" to be evacuated, the symptoms would have been brief and mild. They were "treated" because they were not. This means that someone with a history of medical treatment for illnesses is inevitably carrying a heavy load of toxins. In the long run, this can lead to "iatrogenic" disorders, medicine-induced illnesses.

The newcomer may be surprised to come down with a cold for no apparent reason. This is a detoxination program; he should leave the medicine cabinet shut. He should NOT drink hot rum toddies, he should drink water. He should NOT drink orange juice that produces no alliesthetic (taste-change) protection against excess. Unneeded substances will only increase the amount of toxic material the "cold" must eliminate; they will amplify the symptoms.

Detoxination symptoms may be relatively severe for a newcomer because of his recent nutritional past. If he lets the program run its course, he will discover that once he has spontaneously recovered, he will clearly *feel better than before he was sick.*

He will also discover that when and if he again has a cold, it is likely to be so mild he hardly notices it.

A long-time Anopsological eater can give himself a two-minute cold on demand. He need only eat an ice-cream cone, and within minutes will have a runny nose . . . for a minute or two. His Anopsological diet will have made him "allergic" to ice cream — only by now, he knows he's "allergic" to *any* unnatural molecules, and that the very notion of "allergy" wouldn't exist but for the assumption that unnatural foods are "natural."

This suggests why people "catch colds" in cold weather: a drop in temperature does the same thing to molecules in the body that it does to molecular bondings in clouds. Cooling slows down the interatomic activity, so that fewer atoms can juggle a toe-hold in the cloud and those that don't "precipitate" out.

As toxins pass through the blood stream on their way out, they may amplify preexisting symptoms. Persons with fungus or "yeast" infections (such as vaginal Candidiasis), or eczema, for example, may experience a temporary "crisis." The reason is that the fungal microorganisms involved thrive on *denatured* sugars that were present in the "normal" diet, which are now being driven out of the body. The infectious agents are nourished by them, but at the same time these agents play a *useful* role by consuming substances the body would be unable to eliminate without them. *Once detoxination is completed the symptoms will vanish,* sometimes overnight. A detoxination crisis of this type may last a week or possibly longer, but if medicines and unnatural foods are not reintroduced, once the symptoms have vanished they will be gone for good.

Because detoxination occurs via the bloodstream, which irrigates the brain, the new instinctive eater may periodically but temporarily experience a "hung over" feeling, blurred vision, pressure, and aches and pains. He may also go through short periods of anxiety and nervousness, but it should not be cause for alarm. Once the toxins are gone, the symptoms they produced will go, too.

In the past, a person may have taken drugs for the symptoms of detoxination. He would do better to leave them alone, pay close attention to the smells and tastes of his food, and be done with the symptoms once and for all. If he is truly concerned, of course, he should see a doctor, but he should inform his physician of his change of diet — and hope he understands the mechanisms involved.

One thing to do if physical or psychological symptoms become intense is to slow down the detoxination process in a natural way. Instead of eating a particular food until the taste changes to "bad," stop eating when the taste veers to merely "not delicious" any more. By not giving oneself the *full* amount of a food one's senses call for, old mismetabolites will be driven out of the cells and into the bloodstream more slowly. This will quiet the symptoms, but of course the final clearing-up will take longer.

Symptoms are the price we pay for our mistaken nutritional pasts. Is it worth the discomfort? Wouldn't it be simpler to take a pill and be done — for the hour, at least? Each person alone can make that choice. But here, as an indication is a fairly representative schedule of therapeutic results that can be expected when instinctual nutrition is practiced correctly. It should not be construed as a promise or guarantee that this pattern will necessarily apply to any given individual, for each one of us is very different, and may have very different varieties, amounts and qualities of food available to him. Nor is this to be construed as an incitement to abandon medical treatment.

The list is based on studies conducted over several years with more than 1500 persons who showed great improvement or complete relief from their conditions:

One Week

Aerophagia. Constipation. Dyspepsia. Fatigue. Chronic indigestion. Migraine headache. Alcohol and tobacco addiction. Obese persons begin to lose weight at the rate of three to five percent of excess body weight per week. Inflammatory pain usually disappears within a few days, with the exception of some specific organs and mechanically damaged nerves — but some alleviation may be expected almost immediately.

Two Weeks

Asthma. Diabetes — reduction of insulin dosages. Diarrhea. Gastritis. Hemorrhoids. Hypoglycemia. Psychological stress. Sexual impotence.

Three Weeks

Allergies of all types. Arterial hypo- and hyper-tension. Arteriosclerosis. Cellulite (subcutaneous fat begins to disappear in three to five weeks). Cholesterolemia. Cystitis. Dermatoses. Immunity to colds. Salpyngitis. Sinusitis. Diminishing of tremor in Multiple Sclerosis and Parkinson's Disease. Hyperhidrosis. Urticaria.

Four Weeks

Amenorrhea & Dysmenorrhea. Excema. Body odors begin to appear in "healthy" persons. Disappearance of pain in Glaucoma. Parasitic infections terminated (in three to seven weeks). Skin regains elasticity; more youthful appearance. Immunity to infections in cuts and burns, with healing time cut in half.

Five Weeks

Arterial occlusion. Recovery of movement in rheumatoid arthritis. Erythema. First signs of improvement in Lupus Erythmatosus. Psoriasis. Skin ulcers. Peptic ulcer.

Seven Weeks

Immunological system reactivated. Amebiasis. Anemia. Athlete's foot. Cataracts. Herpes Simplex. Immunity to contagious disease, remarkable resistance to fatigue. Leukemia. Proteinuria. Rheumatoid Arthritis.

Twelve Weeks

Baldness: first reappearance of hair. Cancer of the breast. Cancer of the larynx. Other cancerous tumors.[1]

Twenty-five Weeks

Hemophilia coagulation rate normalized. Hyperthyroidism improved. Myasthenia, Multiple Sclerosis: recovery from paralysis, improved balance and coordination.

One Year

Corns disappear. Rapid painless childbirth with amniotic sac breaking at end of process rather than at beginning. Blood Rh-factor incompatibility disappears.

* * *

Many people, doctors included, often assume that an absence of visible pathology is the same thing as "good health." But there are profound differences between a normally fed person's "good health" and someone fed on foods that nature intended. By eating consistently by instinct, one may not only cure or prevent disease, but acquire a state of well-being that goes far beyond what is generally thought of as "normal." Some frequently observed improvements include these:[2]

Nails. For reasons that are not understood, *fingernail and toenail growth slows dramatically.* Frequent trimming becomes unnecessary. Cracking and other nutritional deficiency symptoms disappear.

Hair. Hair has been seen to grow back on mens' bald heads in a few cases. Hair growth is evidently a sign of the body's overall vitality. Under Anopsological conditions hair growth generally increases. Furthermore, hair *color has frequently been seen to return from white or grey hair.*

Resistance to cold. Persons who suffered from cold weather will discover that it no longer bothers them as much. One instinctually nourished man fell into an ice-cold lake and spent the night clinging to his capsized boat before being rescued the next morning. He reported that after about 15 minutes he felt "warm all over," and suffered no after-effects at all from his prolonged immersion (except a need to catch up on lost sleep). Most instinctual eaters report a similar resistance to cold – and animals fed Anopsologically can be seen to tolerate cold weather extremely well.

Resistance to heat. People who were "allergic" to the sun or were easily sunburned will discover that it no longer happens. They will also discover that if and when they burn themselves (e.g., on a stove), the pain disappears almost immediately and does not return, and that no blisters form.

Body odors. For someone who is in generally good health at the outset, body odors — including the odor of your feces and urine — will disappear entirely after a few weeks or months. They will reappear only during a detoxination crisis. However, persons with severe pathology (i.e., cancers, auto-immune disease) will continue to have body odors as long as their conditions persist.

Healing. Healing time for cuts, burns, and bruises, is about half what is generally thought of as "normal." There is no pain after the first few seconds. The same applies to broken bones. One instinctual eater, an amateur mountain climber, was covered with severe bruises after a fall. To his surprise, they disappeared completely in less than three days.

Bleeding. Hemophilia has been cured with Anopsotherapy. Coagulation occurs rapidly even in severe cuts. Menstrual bleeding becomes a barely perceptible flow, free from odors.

Stools. Persons who were previously constipated or suffered from diarrhea will be surprised to discover that their stools have *perfect* consistency, i.e., they will not even leave residues that have to be wiped away, and they will be odorless. Anopsologically fed animals also have odorless stools.

Fatigue. Anyone can expect to increase his stamina and tire much less than before. However, he may be less capable (or willing) than before to fight a need for sleep when he feels it, since he will be more in tune with himself and obedient to his body's demands.

Skin. Skin becomes more elastic, and acquires a rejuvenated appearance. Moles, warts and other blemishes will dry up and disappear after some months.

Nervousness. Instinctive nutrition quiets the nervous system. People are able to face adversity with more inner quiet than they knew before. They can expect to sleep well and to wake up refreshed. They experience a surprising degree of inner peace.

Sexual Potency. Men and women alike report recovery of their sexual interest and capacities. However, it is no longer a compulsive, tension-releasing sexuality as much as a deeper organic sexuality they experience, more satisfying but less frequent. A person will be disappointed if he expects to win sexual marathons thanks to instinctive nutrition.

Childbirth. Instinctively nourished women give birth without pain. Labor may carry intense feelings, but is painless. Once the process has begun, it is completed within a few minutes, on condition the mother is in a sitting or standing position. If she is lying down, the natural process will be arrested. The amniotic sac remains intact until the baby's head has reached the vulva, providing hydraulic protection through the birth canal. The mother is not exhausted, and is able to care for her child at once. There is no danger of infection. In some 35 cases on record, no complications have been observed. This is not to suggest someone plan to have her baby under a tree, but she might consider eating the fruit of that tree, along with other foods *in their original state* as soon as she discovers she's pregnant. However, it may not be a very good idea to *begin* instinctual nutrition after the fifth month since the fetus will have to bear the impact of detoxination occurring via the mother's bloodstream.

Perceptions. The senses of smell and taste become immeasurably more acute. You can expect your hearing and eyesight to improve, except temporarily when detoxination is taking place.

Teeth. With the extraordinary immunological reactivation this nutrition produces, persons can expect to find fillings falling out of their teeth. This is an area where one will have to exercise care, because *dental cavities will normally be painless,* so one may feel no compulsion to have them fixed. But you must have the fillings replaced. Gum problems, however, can be expected to clear up. We should blame our dental problems on our denatured past. Proper nutrition can help many things, but it cannot necessarily rewrite a person's alimentary history.

[1] Cases on record. No one may claim ability to cure another's cancer, but by choosing his foods correctly a person can help himself cure his own.
[2] Anyone will discover most of these things themselves if they practice Anopsology correctly and persistently. If they stick even partially to "normal" nutrition they may not, but they should experience some improvements nevertheless.

Chapter 26

What We Discovered

The effects of instinctive nutrition often sound "too good to be true," until one has experienced them for oneself. But the method works, regardless of age. Testimony to this is borne by the following words of Gertie Bagage, an Irish woman married to a retired French businessman, living in a small town in central France. She asked that her story be included here so that others might have an opportunity to read it and take hope . . .

We'd both been feeling awful for an awfully long time. Maybe it's inevitable in your sixties. My lumbago was permanent. My husband's sciatica was an uninvited guest thrice a year, presumably incurable. He would joke about it all — when he felt good enough to joke. Our cardiologist insisted that gentle exercise — walking for at least an hour a day — and eating greens, were musts if his angina pectoris was not to carry him away. He did nothing but lie on his couch asking for second helpings of *pommes de terre dauphinois* or toast and jelly. It was only when a friend remarked that with his limp and walking stick he looked distinguished "like a retired English colonel" that we finally decided to do something about it. But what?

"Seek and Ye Shall Find," and to make a very long story short, we at long last ended up in a course on Instinctive Nutrition.

What attracted us from the start was the ground-roots simplicity of the thing. Uncomplicated. Logical. Scientifically sound. Not a cult, for a change.

Our first meal was almost frighteningly simple. Here are fruits: smell them one by one. Choose the one that smells best and eat it until it doesn't taste good any more. I resisted it; it went against the grain. But finally, reluctantly, I agreed to play the game. I felt so foolish! I explored; I discovered that the fruit that smelled the best tasted best. I didn't realize it then, but my husband and I had just put our feet on the first rung of an An-op-so-logical ladder . . . I can hardly pronounce it.

The following days were fun — funny fun. It wasn't so much the fruits and nuts, but could I ever have believed I would some day be comparing the odiferous qualities of raw tuna fish and sardines? It had been obvious to me that never in my life would I eat raw fish. And here I was, stunned by the discovery that my mind could only think, while my instinct *knew.*

A day or two later I ate seven bananas — talk about excitement! — I had been allergic to bananas for years! It was about then that I began eliminating my stored-up wastes. I felt vaguely convalescent without having been sick; an afternoon nap became a ritual for a while.

I had been sleeping badly for years, and now I suddenly realized that sleep was coming easily and I was waking up . . . *refreshed!* That was worth all the raw tuna fish in the world. But my dreams were full of food: the tastes, the smells, the sights of food, and cooked food, and wheat fields exploding and burning to ashes. I began to laugh hysterically, and I said this was all too crazy, we couldn't go through life just thinking about food. Oh please, Lord! Hot, roasted, boiled, baked, braised, toasted, grilled, any way at all, but please, Lord, hot instead of raw! I laughed and laughed until I realized I was crying.

I had come to the bridge of asses and fallen off. When I got home I took a tray, my favorite china and crystal and silverware, and I made a cooked meal. The refrigerator was almost empty, but I boiled an egg, toasted some wholegrain bread, made tea and scones with raspberry jelly. My husband didn't want me to sink so low all alone; he prepared a tray for himself. We ate slowly, in religious silence. Then we sat back and passed judgment.

"Not bad, but not as good as I expected" – "me neither."

My husband's next meal was raw oysters, but I had boiled potatoes, and kept eating cooked food for two days. And then I decided: I'm going back to eating it raw. I had been sleeping better, I had been losing weight. I needed to give it a chance. But now I was free to decide because of my excursion back into cooking. I no longer felt trapped in something too big for me. I didn't feel guilty, either. That evening I went back to my instinct.

I kept thinking about cooked food for some time – I now call it my "tight-rope" period. I knew that any time I wanted to I could plunge back into cooked foods. I will? I won't? It seemed like the balance would tilt at the slightest provocation. Why tempt the devil? No dinner invitations sent or accepted . . . until one morning I realized I was thinking about food again – *raw* food!

Our energy simply amazed us. We got thin as rails while eliminating our wastes, then put it all back on as muscle. My husband lost 45 pounds. Our heads were clear, we didn't tire. For me there was time and energy saved as well: no menus to think out, no cooking to do, no dishes except rinsing them, no pots to scrub – I spent only a few minutes a day in the kitchen. Now I *really* understood Women's Lib!

We were eating only what our bodies needed, no useless extras. No hard digestive work to use up energy. Now we had it for other things. It was a little expensive at first, because we were trying to bring the tropics to our table. In time expenses diminished, as our buying know-how improved.

It was at the end of three months that we visited the cardiologist. He could hardly believe it. My husband's blood count was normal. There were no signs of angina. My own blood pressure was back to what it had been at age 20. The doctor's prescription was this:

1)Stop all medication (he had already stopped it about the third day), 2) continue eating this way, 3) exercise within reason.

Nine months have now passed and we're both like new. We've stayed in touch with a few other people who started the "diet" at the same time we did: the 19 year-old girl with leukemia, the 45 year-old woman with cancer, the 50 year-old man with diabetes, the expectant mother, pregnant with her third child, who had been sick for the entire duration of her previous pregnancies — all of them told the same story: improvement after only a few days or a week . . . on the sole condition of eating by instinct.

A few days ago my husband single-handedly moved a bed down a flight of stairs to another room. He didn't complain about not being in shape like he used to be, just the opposite.

— Gertie Bagage

Chapter 27

A Word to Professionals

Anopsotherapy in theory is simple, and many will be tempted not only to use it for themselves, but to coach others and offer them the services of an "Instinctive Eating Place" or "Diet Center." But *unless they have themselves been practicing it correctly for some time* they are likely to make mistakes for which their clients will pay a price. Regularly, neophytes appear who attempt to "improve" on Anopsotherapy by offering food supplements in addition to the food itself, by encouraging the use of foods having a "high fiber" or "low fat" content, by making recommendations that reflect their theoretical biases rather than the patient's biochemical urgings. But in matters of nutrition one cannot "improve" on nature. We have learned to do that in so many other areas, that we are easily tempted to try it here as well.

Undenatured food is difficult to obtain in the marketplace. Therapeutic effectiveness depends on food being truly in its native condition, free of toxins. This is not necessarily critical for someone in fairly good health, but in severe pathology, denatured food can potentially worsen the very condition it was intended to cure. If this happens, both therapist and patient may wish to revert to more familiar techniques, condemning the methodology rather than the food. It is important that both understand the mechanisms involved.

The person setting out to offer instinctive therapy to the public should have mastered the method himself; a purely intellectual understanding of it will not suffice. Only by experiencing the reactions and transformations it produces can one know how to interpret them and explain them to others. A detoxination sequence may carry all the symptoms of a known disease entity, but should the therapist or patient misunderstand the process involved, and call for it to be "treated" with drugs, he will end the patient's chances of truly getting well. On the other hand, it can be dangerous to suddenly suspend previous medication, on the assumption that the organism's instinct and spontaneous self-healing will instantly take its place. In most cases it will – but only with time. The therapist must understand the problems involved in order to correctly guide others.

The therapist should also have other essential knowledge. He should understand the use of taste intensity, attraction and revulsion as a therapeutic tool, the meaning of body odors, the role of fever, the significance of temporary symptom reappearance, and how dietary exceptions produce symptoms. He should also understand how cultural values, nutritional theories, old preferences, and dietary addictions among other things, act to distort sense perceptions, and he should be able to help patients overcome them for maximum therapeutic effectiveness.

We want to encourage the use of *Anopson*. But we caution the blind from leading the blind. Those who wish to offer it to the public should first master it correctly themselves.

Chapter 28

Improving Health Even With Denatured Foods

Even with the best of intentions, not everyone can or wants to eat consistently only native foods selected by instinct. Business people on the move may find it particularly difficult. Some see it as a constraint (although once they do it they will find it is the *easiest* way to eat). Others may be psychologically unprepared to give up old ways, or be reluctant even to explore the smells and tastes of raw foods.

It was mentioned earlier that a person's vitality and health will benefit even if instinctive nutrition is practiced only in part. Here are a few suggestions about how to do this – how to use Anopsological principles to good advantage with a "normal" dietary lifestyle.

One vital and fundamental point should be kept in mind: *our human biochemistry is genetically programmed to process correctly only the chemical compounds in foods found in nature.* Our bodies cannot properly use denatured or unnatural (for humans) foods. What this means, in *any* nutritional setting is:

1. *the more natural (raw) foods one eats, the better off one will be, and*

2. *the fewer unnatural foods one ingests, the better off one will be.*

Instinctive nutrition implies the total elimination of unnatural substances, and this is what enables a person's body to progressively cleanse itself of accumulated toxins, and obtain the nutrients that will produce the benefits mentioned earlier. Short of that, however, one can receive *some* benefit, at least, by simply *reducing toxic input.* This can be done most effectively by first excluding the most toxic foods from one's diet, while keeping everything else. Later one can eliminate other foods that are relatively less toxic, and progress in stages toward an entirely toxin-free instinctive regime if one decides to go that far.

Earlier I discussed which foods are truly natural for humans, and how they are most often denatured. From this it should be clear that as a general rule, the most toxic foods will be those that both 1) are not native foods for humans in the first place and 2) have been further denatured by high temperatures.

Consequently, the single most important class of foods one should do without is: *cooked (pasteurized) dairy products.* This includes whole milk, skim milk, buttermilk, lactose-free milk, condensed milk, powdered milk, cream, cheese, butter, ice cream, yogurt, cottage cheese and any and every mixture containing dairy products in any form or amount. There is no reason for human beings to suffer nutritional deficiencies without milk because *milk is not a native food for humans to begin with.*

Step 1 for Toxin-Reduction: Completely Do Away with Dairy Products.

Doing away *completely* with dairy products will enable the immune system to become intolerant of mismetabolized milk residues in the organism and clean them out. If a person stops ingesting *all* dairy products initially for two or three weeks, he will probably then discover if he tries one, that it produces an "allergic" reaction (a detoxination event – please see chapters 9 and 10). He will then (but not before) be able to understand what they were doing to him previously.

The second most toxic class of foods after milk is: *baked cereal grains,* and in particular, *wheat.*

> *. . . in Europe during World War II, when wheat imports were reduced by 50% schizophrenic admissions to the mental wards fell by nearly the same percentage. On Formosa, the natives eating very little of the grains are reported to have a schizophrenic rate nearly two-thirds less than that of northern Europe. How many institutionalized schizophrenics might be improving or released to rejoin society, if bread were not the staff of mental hospital diets . . .* [1]

Can "The Staff of Life" really be harmful? It warrants a closer look. Bread is one of the most chemically active mixtures in Western nutrition. This is why:

Batter is made essentially from flour, a powder made by grinding intact ("whole") or partial ("refined") cereal kernels into fine particles. When grains are milled they are haphazardly broken apart. This has the effect of increasing the surface area of the grains with respect to their volume. A single grain might weigh, for instance, 1/10th of a gram, and its surface area might be one square millimeter. Once ground into 100,000 small pieces, let us say, its weight will essentially be unchanged, but its exposed surface area will have increased about *half a million times* (for simplicity's sake, if each particle were a hypothetical perfect cube, its surface area would increase by 50% every time its volume was quartered). In other words, the number of sites where cereal atoms are exposed to each other and to non-cereal atoms is increased phenomenally.

When flour is mixed with other powdered ingredients and fluids it forms a colloidal suspension, in this case a "paste" that clings together because the electrostatic attraction between exposed atoms at the surface of the particles is now so powerful with respect to the size of the particles, that it binds them together (the very same reason why concrete is so solid). This suspension, or dough, is practically impossible to digest, but thanks to gasses and other effects of high temperature during baking, the bonds are weakened and the particles driven far enough apart to be cut with a knife.

Our teeth can cut them apart too, but can our enzymes? The more ingredients there are in a mixture, the greater the molecular variety and interactive complexity. The closer the surface molecules are to each other, and the higher the temperature, the more compounding there will be. The final product is something else entirely than the simple sum of the original components.

To speak only of the cereals themselves (disregarding for a moment what was done to them) — they were not a major food for humans in the first place, not a native food at all when ungerminated. The smell and taste of practically any germinated cereal may occasionally become attractive, like any other natural product that fills a nutritional need. But we know now that instinctive eaters are regularly attracted to only *minute* amounts of any germinated cereal before its taste turns bad — rarely more than a few mouthfuls (hardly as much as might go into a single slice of bread). And since an unnatural *amount* of a food, greater than that demanded by instinct, can be just as toxic as an unnatural *kind*, it shows what one needs to do about bread:

The less the better.

And toasting only denatures it further.

Step 2 for Toxin Reduction: Avoid Baked Cereal Mixtures.

Another highly toxic type of food is *mixtures cooked at high temperatures*. A food that was natural when raw will become unnatural when cooked (please see chapter 4). When foods, even native ones, are mixed together at high temperature, they produce thousands of novel chemical compounds that our biochemistry does not know how to process, that in the long run will make us sick. As a general rule, the more complex the mixture (the recipe), and the higher the temperature, the more toxic it will be. (Note also that the higher the temperature, the more a food's nutritional value is destroyed.)

Since low temperatures produce fewer new chemical compounds than high ones, and fewer ingredients provide fewer sources for aberrant molecular recombinations, this simple principle should be anyone's guide for cooking:

Keep it simple, keep it cool.

Steaming (in an unpressurized vessel) should be preferred over boiling, boiling over baking or frying. If foods are fried or baked, they should be done so *slowly*, with the heat kept as low as possible. If food is cooked over an open flame or coals, it should be kept as far away as possible, and cooked for the shortest possible time. Pressure cookers should be avoided because they shorten cooking time by raising the temperature, which produces more novel compounds than an open pot.

Cooked mixtures should be kept to the lowest possible number of separate ingredients. Seasoning should be added after cooking, not during it or before. Stews, soups, and sauces should be kept as simple as possible, or avoided entirely if possible. Canned or dehydrated preparations should be avoided entirely.

Step 3 for Toxin Reduction: Few Ingredients, Low Temperature.

The reader may wonder, if I follow these guidelines, will it leave me with anything at all I can benefit from and yet still enjoy? The answer is, it will *increase the attractiveness of truly beneficial foods* because as body intoxination diminishes, the senses will find simple foods, and particularly raw foods – *real* foods – more pleasurable. For example, former bread eaters will discover more pleasure with fruits than ever before. Former milk drinkers will discover new gastronomic satisfactions with almost every kind of original food.

The outcome will be better health, more vitality, a happier and perhaps longer life.

In Summary:

FIRST ELIMINATE DAIRY PRODUCTS *COMPLETELY*
THEN LITTLE BY LITTLE
STOP EATING BAKED CEREAL PRODUCTS
AND
COOK WITH FEWER INGREDIENTS AT LOWER
TEMPERATURES

These simple rules, which can serve as a guide in restaurants as well as at home, should help you feel better than ever before. Once that happens, you may want to go even further toward the kind of pain-free, disease-free health that instinctive nutrition makes possible. When you're ready to, reread the how-to part of this book . . . and then *DO IT.*

Carlton Fredericks, *Psycho-Nutrition*, Grosset & Dunlap, New York, 1976., p. 85.

For Further Information

Instinctive Nutrition Center
6 Hurndale Avenue
Toronto, Ontario M4K 1R5
Canada

North American information clearinghouse and networking center for instinctive nutrition and therapy. Offers a seminar and retreat program in cooperation with local organizations.

Centre National d'Anopsologie
Chateau de Montramé
77650 Soisy-Bouy — France
Phone: 1 64 00 26 10

The French Anopsology center near Paris. Maintains an ongoing educational and therapeutic program in a medieval chateau setting, with rustic comforts and superlative food quality. Some staff members speak English.

Information (in English) available in the U.S. through the Instinctive Nutrition Information Center.

"Les Fontanilles"
66300 Maureillas — France
Phone: 68 83 08 11

This small family-operated instinctotherapy center near Perpignan in southern France offers simple but clean accommodations in a quiet mountain setting, with a good variety of high quality foods in a home-like atmosphere. Information available through the Instinctive Nutrition Information Center.

Bibliographical References

In addition to the material referenced in footnotes, the following works may prove helpful to readers wishing to explore further the field of Anopsology and the orientations it implies.

ALEXANDER, F. Mathias, *Man's Supreme Inheritance*, Re-educational Publications, Ltd., London, 4th Ed. 1957.
Shows how preconceived ideas and stereotyped attitudes stand in the way of organic harmony. Important for persons who have difficulty trusting their senses.

BURGER, Guy-Claude, *La Guerre du Cru*, Roger Faloci, Paris, 1985.
In French, a philosophically provocative and amusingly illustrated introduction to Anopsology, in the form of a Socratic dialogue, by the man who first put it into practice.

CLARKE, Robert, *Naissance de l'Homme*, Editions du Seuil, Paris, 1980.
In French, a study of the development of civilization, and most importantly in the context of Anopsology, of agriculture and animal husbandry.

HOWELL, Edward, *Enzyme Nutrition*, Avery Publishing Group, Wayne, NJ, 1985.
A vital and fundamental work that explains why raw foods are, in effect, the only foods humans should eat — and how the cooking of food may be the cause of all humanity's bodily ills. Although already referenced, this book is listed here to emphasize its importance.

JANOV, Arthur, *Primal Man*, Thomas Crowell Co., New York, 1975.
— *Imprints*, Coward-McCann, Inc., New York, 1983.
These works by the creator of Primal Therapy, explore Primal mechanisms in man and show how the effects of prototypical (including chemical) events may remain active throughout a lifetime.

JASTROW, Robert, *The Enchanted Loom*, Simon & Schuster, New York, 1981.
A study of the evolution of brain structures and "intelligence" from earliest times to present. Conveys a feeling for the working of evolutionary processes.

KORZYBSKI, Alfred, *Science and Sanity, An Introduction to Non-Aristotelian Systems and General Semantics*, The Institute of General Semantics, Baltimore, 4th Ed., 1980.
Perhaps the most important book of our time for understanding the mechanisms of human knowledge and the role of unconscious assumptions. Should be required reading for anyone claiming status as a "scientist."

PERLES, Catherine, *Prehistoire du Feu*, Masson, Paris, 1977.
In French, the "Prehistory of Fire," a study of its earliest known use by men.

PERLS, Frederick S., *Ego, Hunger and Aggression*, Vintage Books, 1969.
  This early work by the creator of Gestalt Therapy illustrates, among other things, how attitudes toward food carry over to other areas...and vice-versa.

SWANSON, Margerie, *Lectures on Electro-Colloidal Structures*, Institute of General Semantics, Lakeville CT, 1959.
  An extraordinary presentation enabling the non-biochemist to grasp some of the complex interactive submicroscopic processes involved in the workings of the organism as-a-whole.

Epilogue

Food for AIDS

This chapter is being included as a postscript because it concerns two patients that could be reported on only after the manuscript of this book had already been sent to the publisher.

It cannot be claimed on the basis of these cases that Anopsotherapy provides a cure for AIDS. But there is little doubt that this method is the most effective available to a carrier of the AIDS virus for delaying if not permanently preventing the collapse of his immune defenses.

There are essentially three stages defined for AIDS: 1) the patient is a proven carrier of the virus but shows no symptoms; 2) the patient is suffering from a variety of infections that can more or less be kept under control by medical means; and 3) the patient's immune system collapses, leading to death from infection.

The two young men whose case histories follow both began Anopsotherapy with AIDS in stage two.

*   *   *

Louis was 25 when he began Anopsotherapy in February 1986. He had been classified as a stage 2 AIDS victim, was suffering from chronic diarrhea, severe weight loss, intense fatigue, asthenia, swollen lymph glands, and exceptionally low lymphocyte levels. And he was desperate.

Three months after beginning Anopsotherapy, following a week of 104° fever with no other symptoms, Louis began to recover. In the space of less than two months his weight became normal, his diarrhea disappeared, his glands became normal, and his lymphocytes were back to normal levels.

Louis went back to his job late that summer. In November he began to have problems at work, became emotionally upset and became increasingly careless in his practice of instinctive nutrition, even reverting to dairy products. His blood platelets fell to 2,000, he was given Immunoglobulin treatment, strict Anopsotherapeutic supervision, and started psychotherapy. By February his platelet level was up to 15,000 (his lymphocytes had not decreased).

Louis is currently under surveillance as an outpatient in the specialized AIDS department of a major Paris hospital, where he has been reclassified as a stage 1 AIDS patient. Since recovering from his relapse his health has been excellent.

*   *   *

Henri was 24 years old when he began Instinctotherapy in September, 1986. At that time he had severe, suppurating acne on face, chest and back, his lymph glands were swollen, his lymphocyte levels were extremely low, he was sleepless, emaciated and chronically fatigued.

He was put on a strict Anopsological regime, no dietary exceptions allowed, and started in psychotherapy. By mid December 90% of his lesions had healed, and his glands were practically normal. By February, 1987 his T lymphocytes were back to normal levels, his glands were normal, and his general health had become, in his physician's words, "excellent."

Henri, who is also under surveillance as an outpatient in the AIDS department of a major Paris hospital, is currently classified as a stage 1, symptom-free AIDS carrier. To this day his health remains excellent.

* * *

There have been others, but none as closely followed as these. To date there has been one recorded failure, a young man named Christian, encouraged by his mother to abandon the nutritional system that had earlier saved him from pneumonia with golden staphylococcus (an event he wrote about in a French homosexual magazine). Then he gave up instinctive nutrition, and died in the fall of 1986 with a stomach full of strawberry cream tarts.

* * *

Here as with other diseases, it should be clear that the AIDS virus is not the sole "cause" of the symptoms, because like other infectious agents, it can only take effect in terrain that allows it to do so. But the terrain is composed, in all cases, of little else than whatever served to nourish it. In this time of a growing epidemic without a cure, the medical profession might do well to sit up and take notice of that fact.

— *Severen Schaeffer*
Paris, June 30, 1987